Understanding
Microscopic Colitis

Other books by this author

- Microscopic Colitis (available in English and Spanish)
- **Vitamin D and Autoimmune Disease**
- **Pancreatic Cancer**

Understanding Microscopic Colitis

Wayne Persky

Persky Farms

United States

First published and distributed in the United States of America by:
Persky Farms, 19242 Darrs Creek Rd, Bartlett, TX 76511-4460. Tel.: (1)254-718-1125; Fax: (1)254-527-3682. www.perskyfarms.com

ISBN 978-0-9859772-8-3

Table of Contents

Introduction

In the first edition of the book titled *Microscopic Colitis* (Persky, 2012) the history of the disease and diagnostic methods were discussed. All of the conventional treatment options that were commonly available at the time of publication were discussed. In addition, non-conventional treatment methods that have been found to be helpful by many patients who were unable to resolve their symptoms by using the treatment regimens prescribed by their physician, were also discussed. Non-conventional treatment methods also tend to be chosen by patients who prefer to treat the disease without the use of corticosteroids or other anti-inflammatory medications or immune system suppressants in order to avoid the side effects of those medications and the long-term health risks that are sometimes associated with them.

But as is sometimes the case with many diseases (and especially with inflammatory bowel diseases), complete resolution of symptoms does not always occur. Whether this is due to individual differences in response to treatments, diet cross-contamination, overlooked medications that can trigger microscopic colitis, overlooked food sensitivities in the diet, circumstances beyond their control, or some other issue, some patients are unable to attain satisfactory remission of all their symptoms. Or as so often happens when medications are prescribed as the sole form of treatment (in the absence of proper diet changes), remission may be only temporary.

And of course many patients prefer to avoid the need to take a medication for the rest of their life, since all medications have side effects that can lead to health issues in certain situations. Younger patients especially are reluctant to commit to using a medication for the rest of their life if an alternative treatment is available that has been shown to be both effective and free from undesirable side effects. In the long term, not only are the health risks of the extended use of medications a topic of concern, but so is the huge expense of long-term treatment with most of the medications prescribed to treat an inflammatory bowel disease.

Over five years have passed since the first edition of *Microscopic Colitis* was published. Progress has been made in understanding and treatment of the disease among medical professionals during that period of time, but many clinicians are still using outdated treatment methods. Out in the real world, where many thousands of patients have to live with this disease every day, the wheels of progress don't turn so slowly. Thanks to the Internet and improved communications, a lot of new information has become available to provide additional insight into how the disease develops, why some patients have more severe symptoms, and why some cases are more resistant to conventional treatment methods. In addition, much has been learned about improved methods for treating the disease.

So much additional understanding of microscopic colitis has happened since the first book was published, that it's time to update our knowledge base in the real world. In general, microscopic colitis patients who actively seek better methods for treating the disease continue to be far ahead of the medical community in their understanding of the debilitating social features of the disease and how to better treat the disease in the long run. This book is based on new and additional information that was not available when the first book was published, and in some situations it expands on information that was presented in the first book in order to provide new insight into successful treatment methods. This edition looks at additional situations that might lead to treatment failure in some cases, and it explores ways to overcome those obstacles.

Conventional medical thinking holds that the inflammation associated with microscopic colitis is due to an increased presence of lymphocytes in the epithelial lining of the colon. But in chapter five we shall see that a completely different mode of inflammation may also be involved, and it may be the reason why so many cases do not respond to conventional treatment programs. This association with the disease has previously been overlooked by the medical community. Ways to identify and resolve this problem are also discussed in chapter five.

And of course there have been numerous new medical research discoveries and this book examines how they relate to treatment programs followed by most major medical facilities, in order to provide an up-to-date perspective on the treatment protocols currently followed by most clinicians. In some parts of the world microscopic colitis is still seldom diagnosed. Because of that situation it may still be incorrectly considered to be a rare disease by medical professionals in those locations. This obviously implies that physicians in those locations are not likely to have the advantage of specific knowledge and experience that comes from dealing with the disease on a regular basis. This may limit their options when treating patients. In addition, this may reduce the likelihood that they will actively search for the disease in patients complaining of digestive symptoms typically associated with the disease. Since microscopic colitis can only be diagnosed by examining slides made from biopsy samples taken from the mucosal lining of the colon during a colonoscopy or sigmoidoscopy exam under a microscope, , a perception that the disease is rare will increase the odds that biopsy samples may not be collected, leading to a failure to diagnose the disease.

Accordingly, the basic information discussed in the first book is not included in this book. Only certain concepts from the first book for which additional insight is now available are discussed in this edition. It should be understood that before considering any of the treatment options discussed in this book, the reader should have a good understanding of the information presented in the first book. Without that background knowledge some of the information in this book may not seem complete, or parts of it may be difficult to understand. And obviously, without the treatment information discussed in the first book, this book does not offer a complete set of solutions. Together, the two books present a comprehensive and up-to-date (as of the dates of publication) coverage of microscopic colitis and treatment methods found to be effective not only by mainstream medical professionals, but also by patients who have looked beyond conventional treatment methods.

Because both the clinical symptoms and the treatments for collagenous colitis, lymphocytic colitis, and most of the other variations of the disease are the same or very similar, in this book the term "microscopic colitis" (MC) will be used to refer to all forms of the disease.

The human body is a very sophisticated and complex organism, and it is made up of numerous complex systems designed to work in harmony in order to nurture, protect, and preserve all parts of the body. Some of the discussions in this book involve medical terms (which are defined in the discussions), but because medical research by its very nature tends to involve somewhat complex scientific concepts, it's virtually impossible to completely avoid some level of complexity when describing the details of how various issues affect the body and its subsystems.

However, every effort has been made to describe any medical or scientific terms used in this book in a manner so that anyone can understand what is being discussed, without the need of a medical background. While reading this book, if you do not completely understand all of the details in some of the discussions, that should not prevent you from understanding the basic principles being discussed, nor should it prevent you from benefiting from the information presented here. Sometimes it may be helpful to reread some of the information in order to better understand it. At the end of each chapter there is a brief summary of the most important points, and that summary can be used to better understand the information presented in the chapter.

Because most references used in this book can be found online more conveniently by most readers who are not likely to have a scientific background by using the older style URL format rather than the newer scientific address system using a digital object identifier (DOI), URLs will be used to identify all online references.

The material in this book is a combination of medically-proven facts (backed up by references) and insight based on my own experiences and the experiences of many microscopic colitis patients who have been kind enough to share their experiences of living with the disease on an Internet discussion and support forum for over twelve years. Most of the material is based on medically-proven, peer-reviewed, published research, although other types of reference information is available where applicable. Whenever an opinion or conjecture is included, it is clearly identified as an opinion, unsupported by medical research. The goal of this book is to bring the reader up to speed on the information and recently-published research that appears to matter in regard to understanding microscopic colitis and how to effectively treat the disease.

Chapter 1

Why Do Treatment Programs Sometimes Fail?

MC can affect our mind almost as much as it can affect our body . . . maybe that's the worst part of the disease, but we may not even realize that until after we've lived with the disease for a while.

As anyone who has the disease is well aware, in some cases microscopic colitis is a complex and difficult-to-control disease. In a small percentage of cases, despite hard work to carefully apply treatment programs that work well for others, nothing seems to bring remission. When medical treatments are prescribed, the medications may fail to bring the expected therapeutic response. And when treatments based on diet changes designed to avoid inflammatory foods are used, the diet changes don't always bring remission — at least not as promptly as anticipated. The lack of treatment success may be due to undetected sensitivities to certain foods, supplements, medications, or environmental issues. Or perhaps there are problems with cross-contamination in the diet. But for whatever reason, the treatments don't bring remission. And with any type of treatment, or with a combination of both medical and dietary treatments, there can be vitamin or mineral deficiencies that can limit the effectiveness of the treatment by compromising the natural healing ability of the body.

And to further complicate the issue there can be sensitivities to items such as cosmetic products, hormone replacement therapy treatments, contraceptives, certain chemical odors, heat, high humidity, mold, pollen, and possibly other environmental influences. Certainly not all patients are significantly affected by all of these potential problems, but any of them can prevent remission in many cases. Obviously, avoiding or at least minimizing all of the potential pitfalls in cases where they are a factor can require hard work, constant vigilance, and dedication. But it is certainly doable if the right procedures are followed.

Food sensitivities are closely associated with microscopic colitis.

Many different environmental conditions have been shown to predispose to the development of microscopic colitis, and those conditions are discussed in the first edition. But in order to fully understand the disease, it's necessary to understand why the inflammation associated with the disease is so persistent and how it is actually perpetuated.

In a nutshell, regardless of the health issues that initially trigger MC (and there are numerous known triggers), the inflammation that perpetuates the disease appears to be due to either certain medications or food sensitivities in virtually every case. And even in the cases where medications are the initial cause of the ongoing inflammation, in most cases food sensitivities soon develop. The presence of these food sensitivities can be easily verified by stool tests to detect IgA antibodies to specific foods. They can also be verified by IgA antibody testing of biopsy samples taken from the intestines. IgA antibodies appear to be responsible for the immune system responses that result in the classic inflammation pattern associated with MC.

Few people are born with food sensitivities, although genetics predispose a relatively high percentage of the population to the potential development of food sensitivities. Most food sensitivities seem to develop as a result of digestive issues caused by side effects of medications, infections, parasites, or some other issue that disrupts normal digestion by causing intestinal inflammation. There are two basic types of food sensitivities, and they are distinguished by the type of immune system response they provoke.

Foods that provoke IgE-based reactions are known as food allergies, and foods that provoke IgA-based reactions are considered to be food intolerances.

The term "food sensitivities" includes both food allergies and food intolerances. The differences between food allergies and food intolerances were discussed in detail in chapter 7 of the first edition of *Microscopic Colitis* (Persky, 2012).[1] Basically, IgE-based reactions occur within minutes or even seconds after exposure, and they typically result in classic upper respiratory or skin allergy symptoms. Severe IgE-based reactions involve anaphylactic reactions that can be life-threatening.

IgA-based reactions typically begin several hours after exposure (following ingestion of the food associated with the reaction) and they result in gastrointestinal symptoms such as gas, bloating, nausea, cramps, and diarrhea. With microscopic colitis, we are primarily concerned with food intolerances, so that will be our main focus here.

To understand how food intolerances develop, it's necessary to understand at least some of the basic details of how the digestive system normally functions. The digestive system must supply the body with all of the basic materials needed to repair and replace damaged cells, and cells that have been marked for replacement because of their age. And it has to supply the energy required to accomplish that, in addition to all of the other energy demands by the body. It also has to provide an adequate amount of certain vitamins and minerals that are required in order to facilitate the many chemical and neurological processes that are necessary for normal functioning of various organs and systems.

The digestive system is able to efficiently regulate all of these complex processes because it has its own automatic control system, known as the enteric nervous system. And the enteric nervous system coordinates its operation with the brain, through the central nervous system.

The building blocks used to create new cells in the body are known as amino acids. When proteins are digested, the molecules are broken down into individual amino acids or short strings of amino acids (short peptides). When carbohydrates are digested, they are broken down into simple sugars. Fats are broken down into tiny globules by bile so that they can be digested by lipase enzyme produced by the pancreas.

All food sensitivities (with one exception) are caused by certain proteins.

Therefore it's the digestion of proteins that is of interest here. However there is one exception to this rule. That exception is mammalian meat allergy, which is caused by sensitivity to a sugar found in all mammals except humans, old world monkeys, and the great apes (van Hage, et al., 2013, Nunen, 2015, Allergy Researchers, n.d.).[2,3,4] The sugar is known as galactose-α-1,3-galactose, or simply alpha gal, or α-Gal. The sensitivity is caused by a tick bite, and if a tick bite triggers the condition, the victim becomes allergic to alpha-gal, which implies an allergy to all mammal meat (excluding the 3 exceptions previously noted). And this allergy extends to dairy products, in some cases. But other than this single exception, all food sensitivities are caused by proteins.

In order to be absorbed into the bloodstream, nutrients must be allowed to pass through the inner lining of the intestine.

This lining consists of a single layer of columnar (tall and relatively narrow) cells known as the epithelium. Both the small and large intestine contain an epithelial layer. The epithelium is actually the top of several layers of the intestinal lining known as the mucosa. The second layer is known as the lamina propria, and the third layer is known as the muscularis mucosae. The lamina propria and the muscularis mucosae provide support and resources for the epithelium. For example, the lamina propria contains numerous lymphocytes provided by the immune system to help prevent pathogens from entering the bloodstream. Normally, the density of lymphocytes is less than 10 or 15 per 100 enterocytes. When inflammation is present, that area of the intestine will usually contain over 20 lymphocytes per 100 enterocytes, and this is a diagnostic criterion for lymphocytic colitis.

The epithelium is the critical link in the interface between the food flowing through the digestive system and the rest of the body (via the bloodstream). It's vitally important that the integrity of the epithelial barrier must be maintained because this is where nutrients are allowed to pass into the bloodstream, and this must be done while blocking the passage of pathogens, incompletely digested food, and other foreign items that could cause serious harm if allowed into the bloodstream. The junctions between these epithelial cells are known as the tight junctions and they normally remain tightly closed. As food is digested, and nutrients become available for absorption, the tight junctions open wide enough to allow the passage of nutrients such as amino acids, without allowing undigested molecules or longer chains of amino acids (peptides) to pass through. Peptides are the result of incomplete digestion. They are partially-digested segments of protein molecules, consisting of medium-length or longer strings of amino acids.

But if the tight junctions open too widely, or stay open too long, these peptides and other inappropriate contents of the intestine can pass through. This condition is known as increased intestinal permeability. It's also called leaky gut, and leaky gut is bad news for health in general because it can lead to many miserable symptoms. When leaky gut allows peptides and other foreign matter into the bloodstream, they tend to be transported to various organs and dumped. When they end up in joints, they can cause arthritic-like inflammation and pain. When they end up in various organs they can cause inflammation that interferes with the proper functioning of those organs.

Gluten is a primary cause of leaky gut.

While food allergies can have other origins, the most common cause of food intolerances can be traced to the fact that gluten causes increased intestinal permeability — for everyone, not just for celiacs (Drago et al., 2006).[5] But people who have genes that predispose them to gluten sensitivity tend to experience a greater intestinal permeability problem when exposed to gluten, so they are more likely to develop clinical symptoms, and they are more likely to develop symptoms earlier in life.

Research shows that the opening of the tight junctions is controlled by a protein in the blood known as zonulin, and certain peptides resulting from the incomplete digestion of gluten and glutelin proteins in wheat, rye, and barley promote the production of zonulin (Fasano, 2012).[6] Normally closed, the tight junctions open wider whenever food is digested, so that nutrients in the intestines can be absorbed into the bloodstream to be transported to the cells where they are needed. It is zonulin's job to regulate when and how much the tight junctions open. And it is zonulin's responsibility to ensure that the tight junctions remain closed then they do not need to be open. But repeated exposures to these reactive peptides leads to increased production of zonulin. And as the process is repeated over and over again with virtually every meal, the tight junctions tend to open wider and stay open longer, allowing larger particles and an increasing amount of inappropriate material to enter the bloodstream.

And this problem (increased intestinal permeability) generally exists not only for gluten sensitivity associated with celiac genes, but it's also present with non-celiac gluten sensitivity (Uhde et al., 2016).[7] For decades the medical community mistakenly denied the existence of non-celiac gluten sensitivity. But Uhde et al. (2016) proved that even when celiac disease and wheat allergy are ruled out, many patients still show the markers of gluten sensitivity, including increased intestinal permeability.

When partially-digested chains of amino acids or other particles that are normally excluded are allowed to pass through into the bloodstream, the immune system immediately recognizes that those invaders should not be there. It marks them for destruction and begins to produce antibodies against them. This primes the immune system so that the next time those peptides appear in the blood, antibody production will be stepped up and an assortment of inflammatory agents will be released in an attempt to destroy the invaders.

With repeated exposures, this leads to a condition where anytime that particular protein is identified within the digestive system, an immune system reaction against it is triggered. And once the production of antibodies is triggered, then that particular protein will always provoke an immune system reaction whenever it is ingested, and a reaction will occur regardless of whether or not leaky gut is present at the time. In other words, once a protein is registered as an antigen by the immune system, a reaction will always be initiated as soon as the immune system identifies the protein, even if digestion of the protein is currently proceeding normally, and the tight junctions are functioning normally.

This is part of the adaptive immune system, the same system that provides immunity to a disease in response to a vaccine. A vaccine prompts the immune system to begin producing antibodies against a specific pathogen so that in the future, any exposure to that pathogen will result in a flood of antibodies that promote the release of additional immune system defense mechanisms designed to destroy the pathogen.

Vaccines work because exposures to antigens of this type are normally discrete events. That is to say, an exposure occurs, the immune system launches an attack and destroys the invading bacteria or virus, and that's the end of it.

But if the antigen is part of the diet, then re-exposure will be a frequent or regular occurrence. That means that the immune system is faced with a never-ending job that it was never designed to have to deal with.

This is the essence of what the medical community incorrectly refers to as an autoimmune reaction.

But the problem is that it's not a true autoimmune reaction because a true autoimmune reaction would be provoked by a part of the body itself. The reaction would never end because it would be perpetuated by cells that are always a normal part of the body.

We know that claim is incorrect because that's not what happens when food intolerances are the cause of the reaction. The reaction is against certain proteins in food, and if those proteins are removed from the diet, then the reaction will end as the antibody levels (antibodies to those particular foods) decline.

The lymphocytes (white blood cells) that infiltrate the mucosal lining of the colon in the case of lymphocytic (microscopic) colitis are one example of an immune system response to the production of antibodies. Ingestion of a food that prompts the production of IgA antibodies in the intestine leads to increased lymphocyte infiltration into the mucosal lining of the intestines. The lymphocytes are sent to destroy the perceived threat created by the peptides that are leaking into the bloodstream. But since these white cells are designed to kill pathogens, they are ineffective at destroying the peptides (which are not actually pathogens and are not alive) and the white cells are unable to effectively prevent them from entering the bloodstream.

Lymphocytes cause inflammation (as a normal part of the process of destroying pathogens), but normally this is only a temporary condition because after the pathogens that were the target of the attack have been destroyed, the inflammation fades away as the populations of T cells, cytokines, macrophages, and various other immune system defenses decline and return to normal levels. But when the attack has been triggered because of food intolerances, it can never end, unless diet changes are made to stop the production of antibodies by avoiding the foods that trigger the antibody production. Without diet changes, the pattern of inflammation that causes microscopic colitis is usually repeated with every meal, so it tends to be self-perpetuating.

The same situation exists with drug-induced MC. As long as a drug that promotes the production of antibodies continues to be used, the resulting inflammation will continue to be produced and the clinical symptoms will be perpetuated.

Anti-inflammatory medications may be ineffective against drug-induced MC.

This can occur simply because the level of inflammation resulting from a drug that causes the production of antibodies may be greater than the efficacy of the anti-inflammatory drug used for treatment. Similarly, in some cases anti-inflammatory medications may be unable to overcome the inflammation generated with each meal by inflammatory foods as long as major food intolerances remain in the diet. But in some cases of drug-induced MC, just stopping the use of the medication that causes the inflammation may be sufficient to bring remission without any need for further intervention. Of course that doesn't always work because in many cases of drug-induced MC, food intolerances may be triggered early on.

Just because only proteins can trigger immune system reactions does not mean that other types of food cannot cause digestive system problems.

It's well known that lactose intolerance can cause digestive upset and diarrhea, for example. Lactose is a sugar. But this type of reaction is not caused by an immune system reaction. It's caused by a deficiency of lactase enzyme which is needed in order to digest lactose. Without an adequate supply of lactase enzyme, undigested (or incompletely digested) lactose will pass through the small intestine into the colon, where it will be fermented by bacteria, resulting in gas, bloating, cramping, and diarrhea.

The production of lactase enzyme is compromised whenever the small intestine is inflamed (yes, the small intestine is also often inflamed when MC is active). Lactase may still be produced, but the quantity is insufficient to digest more than small amounts of lactose. This even occurs as a result of the flu, although it is short-lived in that situation. Likewise, if the inflammation continues for longer periods (as with any inflammatory bowel disease), MC patients may also lose the ability to produce normal amounts of other enzymes that are important for the digestion of carbohydrates and sugars.

They may eventuality lose some of their ability to produce enzymes such as amylase, cellulase, invertase (sucrase), peptidase, and malt diastase (maltase). These are sometimes called brush border enzymes because they are found in what is known as the brush border region of the small intestine.

The internal lining of the small intestine is covered with tiny finger-like projections known as villi, and the villi are covered with microvilli to enhance digestion and the absorption process. These microvilli are so small that even under a microscope they appear similar to "hairs" or "brush-like", but under an electron microscope they can be clearly seen. The surface of the villi is comprised of a layer of epitheleial cells. Amino acids and other nutrients, including short-chain peptides, are absorbed into the bloodstream between these epithelial cells,. as discussed earlier in this chapter. As MC patients continue to lose their capacity to produce adequate amounts of certain enzymes, their ability to completely digest certain foods, especially carbohydrates, becomes increasingly difficult.

The ability to produce normal amounts of certain enzymes tends to be lost in a definite order (with respect to the enzymes involved), and as the inflammation is resolved, most of the ability to produce enzymes will be restored in the reverse order in which it was originally lost. Lactase is the first enzyme that will be lost, and it is the last one to be restored after the inflammation ends.

In many cases though, capacity may not be fully restored to the original status. During periods of inflammation, the progressive loss of these enzymes tends to cause increased fermentation (of partially-digested foods), resulting in gas, bloating, and other symptoms that are so familiar to MC patients.

Normal or above-normal amounts of fiber in the diet are contraindicated for MC patients. The mucosal lining of the intestines is already inflamed, and fiber irritates and tears the cells in the mucosa, causing additional inflammation (Eades, 2006, August 30).[8] Minimizing fiber is almost always beneficial when selecting foods for a recovery diet.

Too much sugar in the diet is typically a problem because (as we've already discussed) when the small intestine is inflamed it becomes progressively less capable of producing normal amounts of the enzymes necessary for the digestion of sugars and complex carbs. Artificial sweeteners are a particular problem, and virtually all MC patients seem to react adversely to most artificial sweeteners, especially aspartame.

Spicy seasonings are also typically a problem, not only because they tend to irritate the gut, but also because many types of imported herbal medicinal products and spices have been shown to contain relatively large amounts of undesirable foreign matter of various types (Posadzki, Watson, & Ernst, 2013, Harris, 2013, October 31).[9,10] Because of these contamination and adulteration issues, avoiding herbal supplements during recovery may be prudent.

Stress, diet, and medications inhibit healing.

Normally, in healthy people the epithelial cells of the small intestine are continuously renewed every 4–5 days, but that schedule may be compromised with an inflammatory bowel disease (IBD). It's well documented that corticosteroids inhibit healing, but published research shows that there is evidence that the combination of conventional diet and lifestyle choices, overuse of medications in general, and increasing stress levels tend to overstimulate the immune system on a chronic level, and this interferes with healing (Bosma-den Boer, van Wetten, & Pruimboom, 2012).[11] The immune system was designed to deal with short-term hazards routinely faced in daily living, issues that could be dealt with relatively quickly. It was not designed to have to deal with chronic problems that can not be completely resolved within a reasonable amount of time. For most people living in today's complex world, the combination of lifestyle demands, health issues, and the associated chronic stress forces the immune system into a state of constant activity. It cannot complete one project before another urgent issue demands attention.

According to Bosma-den Boer, van Wetten, and Pruimboom (2012) this condition of compromised functioning results in unresolved inflammation, and significantly increases the risk of chronic disease. The odds of modern lifestyles becoming less complex and less stressful anytime soon appear to be extremely slim, so learning effective ways to manage stress of all types will almost surely become increasingly important as a means of safeguarding and enhancing personal health. We'll look at stress in more detail in chapter 7, specifically with regard to how it affects microscopic colitis.

Why do some MC patients have so many food sensitivities?

This appears to happen because when digestion is compromised by the inflammation associated with the disease, many foods are only partially digested. Though the disease is named for its classic colonic inflammation, many other organs in the digestive system also tend to become inflamed. For example, the stomach and small intestine are commonly inflamed (Koskela, 2011).[12] And less frequently, the pancreas may become inflamed, either because of the disease itself, or because of some of the medications used to treat IBDs (Pitchumoni, Rubin, & Das, 2010).[13]

When these organs are inflamed, their ability to produce normal amounts of the enzymes necessary to digest various types of foods, is limited.

And if leaky gut is present, the immune system can be flooded with perceived threats due to all the "foreign" items that can end up in the bloodstream as peptides from incompletely-digested food. As a result, many of those proteins may be labeled by the immune system as antigens, and future exposures to them will provoke an immune system reaction.

So in general, leaky gut is necessary before food sensitivities can develop.

Certain proteins are much more likely than others to provoke an immune system response of this type. But in virtually all instances, before a dietary protein can be marked as an antigen that provokes the production of antibodies, leaky gut must be present. So it appears very likely that every person who has food sensitivities either has leaky gut, or at least has had it in the past (when the food sensitivities were initially developed). So leaky gut is closely associated with microscopic colitis. Of course it's possible to have leaky gut without having MC, but it appears very unlikely that someone could have active MC without having leaky gut.

What actually causes leaky gut?

Virtually all organisms (especially plants) produce chemical compounds that can antagonize the digestive system to cause irritation, inflammation, or even toxicity, when ingested. Because plants evolved with no means for escaping by running or flying away whenever a predator decides to make a meal of them, they have managed to develop antinutrients that can make them much less appealing to certain predatory organisms. Antinutrients are chemical compounds that interfere with the body's ability to absorb essential nutrients. Normally they're not a major concern for most people, but they may become a problem if malnutrition develops because of some other issue. And they may be a problem for someone following a vegan diet, especially if other digestive issues should develop. IBDs fall under the category of "other digestive issues", so antinutrients should certainly be considered as a possible contributor to the inflammation that perpetuates MC.

We are taught from infancy that we should eat a balanced diet that includes a variety of food.

In the United States, most of us grew up under the shadow of the government's (USDA) infamous Food Pyramid, which in my opinion is one of the main reasons why allergies and many diseases are on the increase today. I can still remember being reminded by my teachers of the importance of the "Food Pyramid" back when I was in grade school. The food pyramid recommended vast amounts of grains (carbs) in the diet, moderate amounts of protein, and minimal amounts of fat, especially from animal sources. Our doctors, Hollywood celebrities, and virtually all other health "experts" parroted the same misinformation and hammered it into our brains.

Then came the "whole grain" campaign, to counter the emerging evidence that refined carbs might be a root cause of many rapidly-increasing health issues such as diabetes, cardiovascular disease, hypertension and obesity. So it's no wonder that our diet priorities became so convoluted — our concept of a healthy diet has been corrupted by well-intentioned but misguided health information. That sounds so much better than saying that we've been brainwashed by misinformation from sources that should know better.

As mentioned earlier in this chapter, during an MC flare the intestines are inflamed and the ability of the small intestine to produce normal amounts of the enzymes necessary to digest various sugars and carbs can be severely limited. This can cause partially-digested carbs to pass into the colon, where they are fermented by bacteria, resulting in typical symptoms of MC, such as gas, bloating, and diarrhea.

Contrary to claims arising from "Food Pyramid"-based thinking, carbs are the only nutrient category that humans can safely totally exclude from their diet and still remain perfectly healthy. Our body doesn't actually need carbohydrates in any amount. Protein and fat are essential diet components, but carbs are superfluous. Carbohydrates (and especially grains) are a cheap source of energy, and as is always the case, we get what we pay for. Cheap energy comes with a cost to our long-term health.

If we get most of our energy from protein and fat (rather than carbs), we can avoid those problems. Eating too much protein and fat (in combination) has few disadvantages, and current research verifies that no major consequences are likely (except for improved health), but eating too many carbs has jeopardized the health of millions and millions of people. Protein is essential for healing damaged tissue. Fat is a much safer source of energy than carbs.

So what do carbs have to offer?

They promote the deposition of fat, they disrupt blood sugar regulation and other metabolic processes in the body, and they are loaded with lectins and other antinutrients that not only interfere with digestion and promote inflammation, but some are also capable of causing increased intestinal permeability. And while it's true that many vegetables are generally good, nutritious additions to anyone's diet, they are by no means essential/indispensable for good health. And they are not free of liabilities.

Protein heals, while carbs disrupt healing and promote inflammation.

Too many carbs in the diet can prevent an otherwise well-designed recovery program from working as expected, even when grains are excluded. Both the fiber and the various lectins and antinutrients found in vegetables (and especially in grains) can promote snd perpetuate inflammation if their combined amounts exceed one's tolerance level. So during recovery, generally the smaller the amount of carbs in one's diet, the more likely that remission will be achieved, and the sooner that goal will be reached. From the viewpoint of someone who has active MC, this could summarized as:

> After remission is attained, (and immune system sensitivity in the digestive tract declines) tolerance levels for various antinutrients should generally improve. But during recovery it's almost always helpful to minimize those risks by minimizing the amount of antinutrients in one's diet.

What type of antinutrients are likely to cause problems?

There are many known different types of these defensive mechanisms, but the most notable examples tend to cause symptoms ranging from irritating to toxic. Some of the antinutrients for which research data have been published include (but are not limited to) lectins, chitins, benzoxazinoids, and amylase trypsin inhibitors (ATIs) Because predators (including humans) typically learn to avoid plants that cause obvious symptoms, those plants are usually avoided, or not even considered to be food. It's the plants that cause more subtle or delayed symptoms that tend to be the most troublesome, because the cause of the problem may not be easily recognized.

17

Lectins are a well-known cause of digestive problems.

They can bind to cell membranes and they can cause sugar molecules to stick together, a process known as agglutination (Sullivan, 2016, October 5).[14] Over three decades ago the wheat germ agglutinin (in wheat) was shown to be a lectin (Kolberg, & Sollid, 1985).[15] The agglutinating properties of gluten are what make the molecules in bread dough stick together and allow it to be kneaded. Lectins normally are not affected by gastric acid or digestive enzymes, so they tend to remain undigested. That means that they retain their antagonistic properties while passing through the digestive system. They can bind to cell membranes in intestinal walls, arteries, and organs, resulting in irritation and possible cellular damage.

Do lectins cause leaky gut?

Clearly, because wheat germ agglutinin is a lectin, that implies that at least some lectins can cause leaky gut. Some of the most common sources of lectins are grains, legumes, dairy, and nightshades. And it's probably not a coincidence that the 8 most common allergens (wheat, dairy, soy, eggs, peanuts, tree nuts, fish, and shellfish) contain some of the highest amounts of lectins. Lectins are probably the main reason why a low-carbohydrate diet works so well to prevent heartburn, gastroesophageal reflux disease (GERD), and sometimes other digestive system problems (because a low-carbohydrate diet reduces lectin intake). Fortunately the problems caused by many lectins can often be minimized by proper cooking methods, but some of them cannot be degraded sufficiently by cooking, so they still cause problems for many individuals.

Certain carbohydrates (specifically mono and oligosaccharides) can bind specific lectins and prevent them from attaching to cell membranes (Sullivan, 2016, October 5). N-acetyl-glucosamine (aka N-acetyl-D-glucosamine, GlcNAc, or NAG) is an enzyme occurring naturally in the body. It's the main binding target of wheat lectin. Therefore it seems reasonable to suspect that this may be the reason why glucosamine compounds have the ability to protect cells in cartilage and possibly in the intestines from inflammation damage associated with gluten-induced arthritis. If the lectins bind to a glucosamine supplement, they can't bind to cells in the body. This implies that the arthritis symptoms associated with MC and other IBDs may be reduced by taking an over the counter (OTC) glucosamine product. In practice, many MC patients and others who suffer from gluten-induced arthritis have found that glucosamine does indeed help to relieve joint pains.

The outer shell (exoskeleton) of insects and crustaceans is made of a polymer known as chitin.

Some authorities claim that because chitins consist primarily of long polymers of n-acetyl-glucosamine (the primary binding target of wheat lectin), they are functionally equivalent to wheat gluten (Mercola, (2011, July 5).[16] If that's the case, then foods that contain significant amounts of chitin, such as barley, rye, rice, tomato and potato should cause major digestive problems. And of course barley and rye do indeed cause the same intestinal damage and clinical symptoms as wheat (because they are closely related to wheat).

But for most people (including MC patients) of all the grains, white rice is typically the least likely to cause inflammation or digestive problems. The same cannot be said for brown rice. The difference between brown rice and white rice is primarily in the husk, which is removed from white rice. And of course the husk contains most of the chitin. Tomatoes are not well-tolerated by many MC patients, but this may be because they are actually a citrus fruit, and citrus fruits are not well-tolerated by the majority of MC patients. While potatoes cause digestive problems for some MC patients, many can tolerate potatoes quite well. So in the real world, while chitins may be a problem for some, they may or may not be a category of antinutrients that cause a significant level of digestive problems for most people (or most MC patients).

Do chitins cause leaky gut?

Based on the effects on the digestive system of foods that contain significant amounts of chitin, it appears that the jury is still out, because the food-based evidence appears to be inconclusive. We already know that barley and rye cause leaky gut, but rice, potato and tomato have not been shown to do so.

However, certain pathogenic organisms that sometimes invade the digestive system may be examples of how chitins can cause leaky gut. All pathogenic fungi contain chitin in their cell walls (Lenardon, Munro, & Gow, 2010).[17] The outer wall of the mycelia (roots or feeding tubes) of Candida albicans are made of chitin. And it's well known that Candida roots penetrate the epithelial layer of human intestines. It's also well known that Candida causes leaky gut. So there is no question that certain situations associated with chitins lead to leaky gut.

Sprouted grains are touted by many as beneficial for health.

But Mercola (2011, July 5) warns of the dangers of sprouted grains, pointing out that they contain benzoxazinoids (Bas), known to be a toxin, and sprouted whole wheat contains some of the highest amounts of wheat lectin. While it's true that the cereal grains (including wheat, rye and corn (maize) contain Bas that are utilized as a defensive mechanism primarily against certain insect pests and competing weeds, rye has by far the most potent effect (Makowska, Bakera, & Rakoczy-Trojanowska, 2015).[18] Corn can cause digestive problems for a relatively small percentage of people, but compared with other foods known to cause significant digestive issues, corn appears to rank somewhat low on the overall scale.

Do benzoxazinoids cause leak gut?

While there doesn't appear to be any medical proof that they do, their presence certainly doesn't enhance digestion in any way. And it's possible that the additional stress that they impose on the digestive system, when added to the accumulated issues caused by other antinutrients in the same foods, or in other foods in the diet, may at least contribute to the development of leaky gut.

Do amylase trypsin inhibitors cause leaky gut?

Amylase enzyme is produced and used by the body to digest carbohydrates, and trypsin enzyme is produced and used by the body to digest proteins. It's been known for decades that legumes (including various beans and soy) contain not only lectins, but also inhibitors of amylase and trypsin (Savelkoul, van der Poel, & Tamminga, 1992).[19] But more recent research data published by Junker et al. (2012) has shown an association between wheat amylase trypsin inhibitors and the activation of toll-like receptor 4 (TLR4).[20] TLR4 is known to promote inflammation.

This discovery has prompted renewed interest in the cause of celiac disease. On the Internet there are even blogs claiming that gluten is not the cause of celiac disease. Instead, amylase trypsin inhibitors are claimed to be responsible. At least one blog even claims that celiac disease is due to the selective breeding techniques used half a century ago to create genetic changes in wheat intended to improve pest resistance.

While that sounds like a plausible observation, it totally ignores the history of medicine.

Celiac disease was first described in the medical literature approximately 2,000 years ago, not 50 years ago (Guandalini, 2007, summer. p. 1).[21] In fact, prior to the 1920s, the medical community didn't have the foggiest idea what caused celiac disease, so they had no idea how it should be treated. For a relatively simple disease (gluten sensitivity), with a simple cure (avoid gluten), why has it taken the medical community almost 2,000 years to figure it out, and why are they still not sure they've figured it out?

TLR4 activation has been shown to cause leaky gut.

It has long been known that chronic alcohol exposure causes increased intestinal permeability, and Li et al. (2013) showed that the mechanism by which this occurs is associated with the activation of TLR4.[22]

> *Chronic ethanol treatment significantly elevated blood endotoxin levels, intestinal permeability, and the expression of TLR4 in the ileum and colon. Moreover, ethanol exposure reduced the distribution of phosphorylated occludin in the intestinal epithelium because of PKC activation. In conclusion, chronic ethanol exposure induces a high response of TLR4 to lipopolysaccharide (LPS), and TLR4 increases intestinal permeability through down-regulation of phosphorylated occludin expression in the intestinal epithelial barrier, accompanied by membrane PKC hyperactivity. (p. 459)*

Therefore, amylase trypsin inhibitors promote leaky gut.

So it appears that it's likely that lectins, chitins, benzoxazinoids, amylase trypsin inhibitors, and possibly other antinutrients may play a role in the development of leaky gut. Whether their respective individual effects are major contributors to the development of digestive system disease, or they turn out to be relatively insignificant, remains to be seen. But one thing we know for sure — grains are associated with all of these issues and legumes are associated with the most potent offenders such as lectins and amylase trypsin inhibitors. In view of all the possible ways by which leaky gut can be induced by the foods that most people eat every day, is it any wonder that food sensitivities are so common?

TLR4 has been shown to be associated with IBDs.

The association of amylase trypsin inhibitors with TLR4 activation appears to have special significance for IBD patients. In research data published in 2005, Oostenbrug et al. showed that TLR4 is associated with both Crohn's disease and ulcerative colitis.[23] Using mice that had been genetically modified to overproduce the active form of TLR4 in the epithelium of the intestine, Fukata et al. (2011) showed that this characteristic increased the vulnerability of the mice to chemically-induced colitis.[24] Mice that have been genetically modified to overproduce TLR4 are known as villin-TLR4 mice. Furthermore, Fukata et al. (2011) concluded that the regulation of toll like receptors affects the outcome of both colitis and associated cancers, and therefore it might have potential as a way to help prevent or treat colitis and the cancers that have been shown to be associated with IBDs.

The discovery that amylase tripsin inhibitors provoke the activation of TLR4-based inflammation fully validates non-celiac gluten sensitivity.

Whether the propensity of amylase trypsin inhibitors to activate TLR4 turns out to be the primary mechanism by which wheat promotes the pattern of inflammation known as celiac disease remains to be seen. But regardless of whether or not that's the case, the potential inflammatory effects of not only amylase trypsin inhibitors, but possibly all of the antinutrients discussed here should equally apply to non-celiac gluten sensitivity. Why? Because TLR4 is part of the innate immune system. That makes it an equal opportunity inflammatory agent, independent of the HLA-DQ2 and HLA-DQ8 genes commonly associated with celiac disease. In other words, it's not necessary for the immune system to develop a sensitivity to any foods that provoke a TLR4 response because all humans are born with that sensitivity.

In support of the above claim (about the ability of other antinutrients to provoke an innate immune system response), it should be noted that both lectins and chitins bind to TLR4 (Unitt, & Hornigold, 2011, Koller, Müller-Wiefel, Rupec, Korting, & Ruzicka, 2011).[25,26] This could well be a game-changer for the understanding and treatment of inflammatory bowel diseases and autoimmune diseases in general, because they are all associated with the inflammatory consequences of food sensitivities.

Are inflammatory bowel diseases contagious?

Recent research by Dheer et al. (2016) has shown that increased TLR4 signaling is associated with an increase in the population and translocation of gut bacteria, and an increase in intestinal permeability.[27] The effects on gut bacteria characteristics imply that increased TLR4 activation might provide the mechanism needed to substantiate the long-held theory that IBDs may be the result of a bacterial infection. And it suggests the possibility of infectious transmission.

For decades, the medical community has denied that IBDs may be transmitted from one individual to another, but experience shows that while this is not common, plenty of examples exist to show where more than one member of a household has developed an IBD. With MC, for example, not only are there multiple IBD cases in some households, but there are also examples of cases where the disease appears to have possibly been transmitted from a human to a pet. MC is actually somewhat common in dogs. While appearances can be deceiving, and it's certainly possible that all these cases are merely coincidental, it's worth noting that Dheer et al. (2016) pointed out that:

> *Interestingly, WT mice cohoused with villin-TLR4 mice displayed greater susceptibility to acute colitis than singly housed WT mice did. The results of this study suggest that epithelial TLR4 expression shapes the microbiota and affects the functional properties of the epithelium. The changes in the microbiota induced by increased epithelial TLR4 signaling are transmissible and exacerbate dextran sodium sulfate-induced colitis. Together, our findings imply that host innate immune signaling can modulate intestinal bacteria and ultimately the host's susceptibility to colitis. (p. 798)*

WT mice are "Wild Type" mice (with no genetic modifications). Villin-TLR4 mice are genetically modified to overexpress TLR4, making them highly vulnerable to colitis and the physiological effects of colitis. While not conclusive evidence, this research certainly suggests that susceptibility to colitis, if not the disease itself, may be increased by close contact with someone who doesn't necessarily have colitis, but is highly susceptible to colitis. That potentially opens the door to possible contagious effects, though clearly the risk (if it exists) must be low, otherwise the transmission of IBDs between humans would be common.

Formulating a diet to avoid the effects of the most potent antinutrients can prove to be quite a challenge.

With so many possible sources of inflammation hidden in so many of the foods that have traditionally comprised a major part of most diets, selecting foods to avoid such inflammatory effects can be difficult. And because of individual immune system characteristics, it's very likely that each of us may be affected to different degrees by various antinutrients. This adds another degree of difficulty to the task of selecting foods suitable for a safe recovery diet for MC patients.

In order for a diet to effectively prevent inflammation from being generated with each meal, all significant sources of inflammation must be avoided. This includes not only the foods that cause the immune system to produce antibodies, but there may be antinutrients that produce inflammation for which no antibody tests are available. We can only guess at this point (due to inadequate availability of research data), but antinutrients may be an important reason why some MC patients are unable to achieve remission despite following a very limited diet that would normally bring remission for other MC patients.

Eliminating gluten from the diet is a "no-brainer".

The neolithic period of our evolutionary history is generally considered to be the dawning of agriculture. Chris Kressor points out that before wheat and its relatives became part of the human diet during the neolithic period, diseases such as diabetes, heart disease, and autoimmune diseases in general, were either rare or did not exist at all.[28] Humans were naturally lean and physically fit. Fertility was not a problem. Sleep came easily and diseases such as Alzheimer's and osteoporosis were not known to be a part of growing older. Anthropological (the study of humankind) evidence indicates that this is true So there are good reasons why gluten should be removed from everyone's diet, not just the diets of people who have discovered that they are acutely sensitive to it.

The human diet became much less nutritious when the neolithic period of our evolutionary history began, and that trend has accelerated during the past 50–60 years.

Note that all dairy products are a neolithic food (along with wheat and all other grains, and soy). Humans most definitely do not need any neolithic foods in order maintain good health. The archeological (fossil) records show that in general, when the neolithic period began, the robustness and general health of humans declined significantly. Humans evolved eating a paleo diet. Our paleolithic ancestors were much bigger, stronger, and healthier than all humans who have lived since then. For the most part, all neolithic foods are detrimental to health, regardless of what many health advocates may claim. It shouldn't be surprising that selecting foods for a recovery diet basically involves avoiding neolithic foods.

How can safe foods be selected for a recovery diet?

Because the food and drug sensitivities of individual patients tend to be so different, dietary needs of MC patients can vary widely. A one-size-fits-all diet is virtually impossible to specify. However, utilizing the data available in the archives of a microscopic colitis discussion and support forum that for well over a decade has focused on controlling MC symptoms by dietary changes, facilitates the selection of foods.[29] As most people who are familiar with using the Internet and social media to search for solutions are well aware, shared real-life experiences can offer priceless information that cannot be obtained anywhere else.

Whole foods cooked from scratch with salt as the only seasoning tend to bring remission and healing much more reliably than more complex diets that include commercially processed foods, sauces, or other condiments. A recovery diet should be considered to be medicine, not a gourmet treat. Most MC patients seem to react to certain specific foods, while certain other foods are almost universally tolerated. And of course there are many foods between those extremes that may be safe for many patients, but that is best determined after remission is achieved. If a bad food selection is included in a recovery diet, then recovery may never occur. Obviously then, only foods that very rarely cause problems for anyone should be considered for a recovery diet, and experimenting with any other foods should be postponed until after the digestive system is working normally again.

It's tempting to add variety, but that introduces the risk of adding one or more foods that may defeat the purpose of the diet by preventing remission. Instead of trying to add variety by adding additional foods, keep the food options small and add variety by preparing it in different ways. If turkey is selected as the primary protein source for example, it can be baked, broiled, grilled, fried, ground and eaten as sausage or as patties, or made into soup or stew. The carcass, neck, other leftover parts, and even the feet can be used to make a nutritious homemade broth that can be used for making soup or cooking vegetables. The broth will add additional nutrients that are very beneficial for healing.

All vegetables should be overcooked to facilitate digestion. Most people who have MC can tolerate veggies such as carrots, squash, and sweet potatoes. Broccoli is usually safe, but it can cause gas, so for those who have a problem getting rid of gas, broccoli may not be a good choice. It's necessary to minimize fiber and sugar, so it's safer to go heavy on the meat, and eat small servings of vegetables.

Fruit is typically loaded with both fiber and sugar, and the type of sugar in fruit (fructose) tends to be more difficult to digest, especially when MC is active. In other words, fruit carries the risk of a double whammy, both fiber and sugar, thus a need to minimize fruit in a recovery diet. It's usually not necessary to totally avoid well-cooked fruit, but the amount per serving should typically be minimized. Most MC patients can tolerate bananas, and bananas are the only raw fruit that is generally safe to be included in a recovery diet. However, not everyone can tolerate bananas, so it's not a universally safe choice. And if too many bananas are eaten, it's possible to overdo the fiber.

Typically, the simpler and blander the diet, and the lower the fiber and sugar content, the more likely that recovery will occur, and the more likely that it will occur sooner, rather than later. Recovery diets that avoid all grains and all legumes, have the highest odds of successfully bringing remission. Sugar should be minimized in the diet and all artificial sweeteners (except for stevia-based sweeteners) should be totally avoided. Rice is usually the most likely grain to be safely tolerated, but not everyone can tolerate rice, so this should be kept in mind if the diet does not seem to produce any significant signs of improvement after a reasonable amount of time. If rice is part of the recovery diet, white rice should be used instead of brown rice. White rice has significantly less fiber than brown rice.

The definition of "a reasonable amount of time" for recovery varies by the individual. Some patients will see improvements within a couple of weeks, while others might require 6 months or more for substantial healing to occur. The severity of symptoms does not seem to be closely related to recovery times. Some patients have much more intestinal damage than others, and various other factors (including unknowns) may complicate the issue, so that recovery time can vary widely. A few patients have been known to require a year or more to reach remission.

Some individuals are sensitive to chicken, so turkey is usually a safer choice during recovery. Virtually no one reacts to turkey. Beef is a problem for some, and a small percentage of MC patients cannot tolerate pork. Therefore a much safer choice is lamb, because sensitivity to lamb is extremely rare. That also applies to venison, goose, duck, pheasant, rabbit, quail, and other wild game meats — virtually all MC patients can safely tolerate those meats. And the game animal does not actually have to be wild. The meat of game animals raised on game ranches or farms is typically just as safe as meat from animals that actually roam wild.

Beef seems to be the most likely domesticated meat to cause problems, and for those who are sensitive to beef, bison is also often a problem because these days most bison carry DNA from domestic livestock. This is true because back in the final years of the 19th century, after the U. S. government promoted the extermination of the vast bison herds of the American West in order to force the Indigenous American Indians to submit to surrendering their freedom so that they could be moved onto remote reservations, bison numbers were so low for several decades that many of them cross-bred with domestic cattle. Additionally, bison ranchers occasionally cross-breed bison with domestic cattle in order to counter the adverse health effects of many generations of inbreeding due to small herd size.

Many MC patients are sensitive to the albumen (egg white) in chicken eggs. Some individuals find that they are able to eat eggs from ducks, quail, geese, or turkeys. While this may be an option, it's usually best to wait until after remission is attained before experimenting with alternative types of eggs, rather than to jeopardize the chances of recovery.

30

It's somewhat common for MC patients to react to tuna and salmon, and possibly certain other fish, (not necessarily all fish), but shellfish are usually a safe choice (except when there is a preexisting allergy to them). Quinoa is usually a safe food, but some brands have been known to be cross-contaminated with gluten. That problem can normally be avoided by purchasing a Kosher brand of quinoa.

Are vegetable and fruit powders easier to digest than whole vegetables and fruits?

The main problems with fruits and vegetables is the fiber, fructose, and sugar alcohols. Most MC patients can tolerate small to moderate amounts of certain vegetables and a few fruits, provided that they are peeled (the peel often contains most of the fiber) and over-cooked to make them easier to digest. Carrots, squash, cauliflower, sweet potatoes, and green beans (even though they are a legume) are usually tolerated by most MC patients. Bananas are usually safe, and many patents can tolerate well-cooked (or canned) pears, apples, peaches, etc. Limiting the total quantity consumed is wise because everyone has their own tolerance limit for the amount of fiber, fructose, and sugar alcohols that can be tolerated during recovery.

This issue was discussed on pages 10–11, the small intestine has very limited ability to produce the enzymes needed to digest various carbs (sugars) while it is inflamed. As the inflammation declines and the gut heals, the ability to produce those enzymes slowly returns, though it may not recover sufficiently to be able to allow the production of normal amounts of enzymes. But the healing process tends to be much slower than most people realize. And challenging the digestive system on a regular basis can delay healing.

Powdered vegetables or fruit still contain the same fiber and sugars as real veggies or fruit, so why not eat the real thing and avoid the processing risks? It's almost always better (and much safer) to get one's nutrients from real (whole) foods, the way that nature intended, rather than from highly-processed commercial products.

Similar to substituting duck eggs for chicken eggs, there are other possible options for substitutions for cow's milk.

Many MC patients have considered using sheep or goat's milk in place of cow's milk, especially for cheese. But unfortunately no one has been able to find any safe milk or cheese or any other type of dairy product that comes from any type of cows, goats, or sheep. It's likely that milk from cameloids (camels, alpacas, guannacos, llamas, and vicuñas) would be safe, because they are genetically different from all of the other milk-producing mammals. It's also possible that equine milk (horses, donkeys, asses, zebras, etc.) might be safe, but finding a source of those products is extremely difficult in most parts of the world. Therefore, most MC patients use either coconut milk, almond milk, hemp milk, rice milk, or some other fabricated milk as a substitute for cow's milk.

In many cases, microscopic colitis tends to be a debilitating disease.

One of the issues that virtually no one understands unless they actually have the disease, is how negatively and profoundly microscopic colitis can affect a patient's mindset and quality of life. Because of the unrelenting and dehumanizing symptoms of the disease, dignity, confidence, and self-respect are all held hostage when the disease is active. Ambitious projects and travel plans often have to be put on hold. In difficult cases, regaining control and restoring one's confidence can require a long and difficult struggle, and in some cases remission may continue to be elusive despite hard work and dedication to treatment protocols that have been shown to be effective for other patients.

As many who have the disease have learned by experience, if the symptoms remain uncontrolled, microscopic colitis can be relentless and unforgiving. Living with it tends to be a life-altering challenge that often includes some downright miserable days. It's well known that many different issues that can cause chronic intestinal inflammation can lead to the development of the disease. And unfortunately MC continues to be relatively poorly understood by many mainstream medical professionals. Consequently, when patients do not respond to conventional treatment programs, the reasons for treatment failure are generally unknown. This lack of information can only add to the uncertainty and stress, resulting in additional loss of confidence and fears of the unknown.

Many GI specialists do not have a good understanding of the disease.

Inexperience with the disease, an incorrect assumption that diet does not play a vital role in the inflammation that marks the disease, and a failure to communicate with patients have been the biggest obstacles faced by gastroenterologists in their attempts to treat MC patients. Common sense dictates that diet matters with all IBDs. Just as surely as the quality of the air that's breathed determines the risk of lung disease, the types of food ingested determine inflammation levels in the digestive system.

Yet even today there are many gastroenterologists who still incorrectly believe that diet has little to do with IBDs. Why do they make such an assumption? Apparently simply because when the disease was first described, no researchers had ever bothered to publish any proof that diet does have an affect on inflammation in the digestive system. Even though proof that IBDs can be controlled by diet changes alone has now been published, many gastroenterologists have not corrected their working knowledge, so they continue to make the same mistake.

Many people find it very difficult to stick with a very limited diet.

But variety in a recovery diet is almost always counterproductive. We grow up thinking that as long as we avoid so-called "junk food", the wider the variety of the foods we eat, the healthier we will probably be. We become accustomed to being able to buy a huge variety of foods, virtually all of which are available year-round. But this wasn't always the case. Prior to about a hundred years ago, food selections were much more limited. And even a couple of generations ago, our grandparents and great grandparents had far less variety in their diet than is available today.

Our paleolithic ancestors ate whatever they could kill, catch, trap, find on trees or bushes, or dig up from the ground. Most tribes ate the same basic foods that were indigenous to the area, which sometimes varied by the season of the year. In some areas, that amounted to a very limited selection of foods. During droughts or other hard times, selections could be extremely limited.

Our early neolithic period ancestors typically ate a very limited selection of foods due to the scarcity of wild game and the monoculture characteristics that dominated agriculture as it was first developed. And this pattern continued for most people for thousands of years. The primitive societies that survived in the wild as hunter-gatherers until a century or two ago typically ate a diet with very limited variety.

Early on, making such dramatic diet changes seems challenging and unappealing.

Adjusting to the necessary lifestyle changes can be tough, especially because little incentive exists on a social level for making those changes. Instead, it's common to feel coerced into making those changes just to satisfy the demands of one's body. This can create an unpleasant atmosphere of resentment of one's own body. We (perhaps subconsciously) may blame our body for trying to destroy our social life.

Explaining to friends and relatives over and over again the reasons why we cannot join them for meals at many of the restaurants where we used to enjoy getting together for an enjoyable meal tends to be embarrassing and frustrating. We may feel that we are being held hostage by our own body, because of the disease.

But the human body is very resilient and it soon adapts to changes. What once seemed strange and difficult eventually becomes normal and routine. And the positive reinforcement that results from feeling so much better due to the diet changes helps to create the incentive needed for sticking with a healing diet.

When starting an elimination diet, the choice must be made whether to cut out all likely food sensitivities right from the start, or just eliminate gluten and dairy and then cut out additional foods later, if necessary. There are obvious advantages and disadvantages to both options, but the primary differences are that simply avoiding gluten and dairy at first is much easier than adopting a complete elimination diet, and this is balanced against a significantly lower chance of successfully achieving remission sooner.

Either method can be successfully used however, as long as one doesn't become discouraged when various dietary approaches fail. The biggest problem with avoiding only gluten and dairy is that it's easy to make the major mistake of assuming that since avoiding those two foods for a few weeks didn't bring remission, then sensitivity to them must not be a problem (when in fact it is).

Avoid falling into that trap, because you may never achieve remission if you allow yourself to make that mistake. It's OK to begin your diet that way, but once you start avoiding a food, never, ever add it back into your diet, or it will confound your efforts from there on out, if you happen to be sensitive to it. This is because as long as you are still reacting, it's impossible for you to be able to tell whether or not you are sensitive to a food being tested unless the reaction stops. As long as a reaction continues, you have no way of knowing. Remember that we can only achieve stable remission if we remove *all* foods from our diet that cause our immune system to produce antibodies.

So if you choose to go that route, until remission is achieved you must continue to remove foods from your diet, but never add any food back in until after you have been in stable remission for a while. After you are in remission, then you can retest the foods that you eliminated to see if you are actually sensitive to them. That usually makes the full elimination diet a faster route to remission, since it bypasses all or most of the experimentation.

Some people who adopt a restricted diet complain of hunger and declining weight.

They remove foods from their diet but continue to eat approximately the same serving size of the foods that remain in their diet. It's easy to forget that as we remove foods from the diet, it's necessary to eat larger servings of the fewer foods that remain in the diet in order to maintain a similar caloric intake. In other words, in order to prevent weight loss, calorie intake must be maintained by simply eating more of the foods known to be safe in order to replace the calories lost due to the diet restrictions.

If maintaining weight or gaining weight is a priority, then avoiding foods that provide no significant amount of nutrition, such as so-called resistant starches may be helpful. Resistant starches pass through the small intestine mostly or totally undigested. When they reach the colon they are fermented by bacteria. The byproducts of fermentation are typically gas and possible bloating. When MC is active, fermentation can also cause cramps and diarrhea. And if any nutrients are made available by the fermentation process, typically they will only benefit the bacteria because most nutrient absorption takes place in the small intestine. In general, only water and electrolytes are recycled in the colon, so foods that are fermented in the colon offer little benefit, especially when MC is active. Foods that benefit gut bacteria are generally considered to be prebiotics, but similar to probiotics, prebiotics are often counterproductive for MC patients during recovery.

It's important to always start the day with a good, safe, high protein breakfast.

Active microscopic colitis sometimes makes eating breakfast difficult or even impossible. But eating a good breakfast will help to provide the protein necessary for healing, and the energy necessary for meeting the challenges that the day may bring.

The timing of meals matters, and in fact timing matters a great deal, according to published research. According to a statement from the American Heart Association (AHA), the timing and frequency of meals have a significant effect on the risks of developing many major diseases and health issues ranging from insulin resistance and obesity to heart attack or stroke.[30] The AHA statement reveals that people tend to eat more snacks today, and they are more likely to eat at different times compared with 40 years ago. That said, MC patients typically find that eating smaller and more frequent meals helps digestion during recovery.

The AHA statement also points out that skipping breakfast increases the risk of heart attack by 27 %, and increases the risk of stroke by 18 %. A prospective study of men aged 40–75 at the beginning of the study showed that skipping breakfast increased the risk of developing type 2 diabetes by 21 % (Mekary et al., 2012).[31] A similar study by Mekary et al. (2013), based on women with an average age of 64.7 years at the beginning of the study found that the risk of developing type 2 diabetes increased by 28 % if they skipped breakfast only once per week.[32]

In a study of Japanese workers between the age of 35 and 66 at the start of the study, Uemura et al. (2015) showed that compared with those who ate breakfast 6 or 7 days per week, those who skipped breakfast more than 2 days each week had a 73 % increased risk of developing diabetes.[33] Odegaard et al. (2013) studied a group of younger people aged 18 to 30 at the beginning of the study and found that those who ate breakfast daily had only 66 % of the diabetes risk of those who did not eat breakfast regularly.[34]

Because microscopic colitis is commonly associated with the development of additional autoimmune diseases, it's probably prudent to take advantage of recommendations such as those found in the AHA statement in order to minimize the risk of developing AI diseases. Beginning each day with a good breakfast is consistent with the research on which those recommendations are based.

It should be noted that the AHA recommends limiting eating to three regular meals each day (to reduce obesity risk). But for many MC patients, the risk of obesity is the farthest thing from their minds. Data based on the accumulated experiences of members of the Discussion and Support Forum for Collagenous Colitis, Lymphocytic Colitis, Microscopic Colitis, Mastocytic Enterocolitis, and Related Issues, shows that eating smaller meals more frequently during the day can improve digestion during the recovery phase of MC. This is because as previously mentioned, when the small intestine is inflamed, (as is the case with many MC patients), enzyme production tends to be limited (Koskela,

2011). With smaller meal size, the digestive system is less likely to run out of the enzymes needed for digesting the amount of food contained in the meal.

Research shows that eating protein with every meal helps to preserve muscle mass as we age.

Rather than to eat most or all of the day's total allotment of protein at the evening meal as many people customarily do, researchers have found that dividing up the total amount of protein among all meals, including breakfast, allows older people to reduce the normal loss of muscle mass due to aging (Mozes, 2017, August 3).[35]

Fasting.

Some patients experiment with fasting as a way to reduce diarrhea when they need to be out and about. But when one has secretory diarrhea, as many MC patients do, fasting does not work so well because with secretory diarrhea water is infused into the colon rather than it being removed (as it would be normally), which means that the diarrhea will continue until the body is completely dehydrated in most cases, which of course is a very dangerous condition.

Nevertheless, it's true that fasting can have health advantages in some situations. For example, studies have shown that those who fast regularly were only about two-thirds as likely to have coronary artery disease as those who did not fast.[36] And patients in this group or a similar group who fasted regularly were only slightly more than half as likely to develop diabetes mellitus. Note that this research appears to contradict the claims made by the American Heart Association and others, as discussed on the two preceding pages.

Similar studies have been published showing that men who ate 4 or more times each day are about half as likely to be obese as those who ate

3 or fewer times each day (Ma et al., 2003, Holmbäck, Ericson, Gullberg, & Wirfält, 2010).[37, 38] Many trials have been published showing that intermittent fasting can be used for weight loss (Harvie er al., 2011, Heilbronn, Smith, Martin, Anton, & Ravussin, 2005, Eshghinia, & Mohammadzadeh, 2013, Johnson et al., 2007, Varady, Bhutani, Church, & Klempel, 2009, Klempel, Kroeger, & Varady, 2013, Hoddy et al., 2014, Bhutani, Klempel, Kroeger, Trepanowski, & Varady, 2013, Varady et al., 2013, Klempel, Kroeger, Bhutani, Trepanowski, & Varady, 2012).[39, 40, 41, 42, 43, 44, 45, 46, 47, 48]

But so far no trials have been done to show that fasting is beneficial for most MC patients, except of course those who are overweight. So while fasting may seem to slow down the diarrhea so common to MC, it usually will not completely stop it until a state of serious dehydration is reached. As long as any free water remains, the diarrhea will continue if secretory diarrhea (watery diarrhea) is the prevailing form of diarrhea, whether the patient eats or drinks anything or not. That said, fasting may reduce the number of trips to the bathroom when other types of diarrhea are present.

What if your gastroenterologist says you need another colonoscopy?

Aside from a colonoscopy given as part of a screening program for colon cancer, usually a request for another colonoscopy is a sign that the patient didn't respond to the prescribed treatment for MC and so the specialist doubts the diagnosis. But MC is almost never misdiagnosed. It is often missed, and the diagnosis will incorrectly be assumed to be IBS in many cases, but you can safely bet that a diagnosis of MC is absolutely correct.

Rather than a case that doesn't respond to conventional treatment being an incorrect diagnosis, the problem is usually that the gastroenterologist simply may not understand the disease, or how to correctly treat it. Some cases respond to the prescribed drugs. But some cases fail to respond because the anti-inflammatory drugs by themselves are not able to overcome the inflammation unless certain inflammatory foods are also removed from the diet.

Failure to understand how food sensitivities are connected with the perpetuation of the inflammation means that a specialist will only be able to treat simple cases that respond readily to anti-inflammatory drugs. The bottom line is that a gastroenterologist who requests another colonoscopy because she or he believes that a patient was misdiagnosed, or has some other problem in addition to MC, often doesn't understand the disease very well.

A repeat colonoscopy will almost always be a waste of time and money for the patient — the patent will undergo the invasive and somewhat risky procedure for nothing, but the gastroenterologist will believe that there's good reason for the repeat procedure. And of course the reimbursement is the same whether a colonoscopy is actually needed, or not.

A dual diagnosis of both CC and LC has little significance in the real world.

Although many patients and GI specialists are concerned that the disease is more severe when the patient is diagnosed with both LC and CC, this actually is a common condition. Many CC patients have the diagnostic markers of LC in addition to the thickened collagen bands (present only with CC), so the opportunity to receive a dual diagnosis is actually a rather common situation.

If a patient meets the diagnostic criteria of CC, it may mean that she or he has had the disease longer. And while the diagnostic markers may be different, the basic pattern of inflammation remains the same, namely above-normal levels of lymphocytic infiltration. The CC diagnosis simply refers to an increased thickness of collagen bands in the lamina propria layer of the epithelial lining of the colon. Some patients qualify for a diagnosis of CC and some don't, but despite the additional diagnostic markers, the clinical symptoms are the same and the treatment is the same.

The confusion may originate when the pathologist notes the existence of the markers of both LC and CC on the pathology report and the gastroenterologist interprets that to imply that the patient has both forms of the disease. The diagnosis is actually CC — the LC is usually implied when both forms of the disease are noted on the pathology report. The reality is that the disease has the capacity to segue back and forth between the two forms of the disease in a seemingly random fashion as time passes. The actual diagnostic markers may vary at the moment at which the colonoscopy is done, but this does not change the clinical symptoms, nor does it change the the indicated treatment.

What if a treatment program fails to bring remission or even an indication of improvement?

There's a reason for everything that happens. The catch of course is that determining that reason is often not easy. And even if the reason for failure can be determined, the problem with a failed treatment program is that treatment must be restarted, or at least redesigned in order to resolve the problem and produce results.

When designing an initial treatment program, rather than to risk going through a series of failed treatment attempts, it's virtually always advantageous to err on the side of caution in order to minimize the odds of failure. Not only does a failed treatment impose additional physical stress on the body because of unresolved symptoms, but the added mental stress resulting from discouraging results imposes a significant additional obstacle to recovery. And of course added stress is the last thing anyone needs when they have a disease that can be triggered by chronic stress.

The advantages of maximizing the odds that a treatment program will be successful should be obvious. So whether an initial treatment program is being planned, or it becomes necessary to refine a treatment program in order to make a second or third attempt to achieve remission, planning for success at every step of the way almost always pays dividends in the long run. Taking extra care to do everything right often prevents having to go through the process again.

Why are corticosteroid medications so effective at helping to reduce the inflammation and thereby helping to control the symptoms of IBDs?

The correct answer to that question can provide some clues needed to help design an optimum treatment program. When physicians prescribe an anti-inflammatory medication such as a corticosteroid to treat MC or some other IBD, they do so because they understand that the drug will help to suppress inflammation.

If the prescription fails to bring relief to the patient however, the reason for the failure will usually be unknown because the mechanism by which corticosteroids suppress inflammation does not appear to be widely understood by most medical professionals. But a search of the medical literature shows that the way in which corticosteroids provide relief from inflammation was discovered and published over 25 years ago (Goldsmith et al., 1990).[49] Based on that research it can be concluded that corticosteroids suppress inflammation in inflammatory bowel disease by reducing mast cell numbers.

Understanding Microscopic Colitis

Later research by Hidalgo et al. (2011) showed that glucocorticoids increase the expression of vitamin D receptors (VDRs), suggesting that vitamin D may actually be responsible for the suppression of inflammation.[50] Corticosteroids (which includes the glucocorticoids of course) may indirectly suppress inflammation by exploiting the inflammation suppression attributes of the active form of vitamin D (by increasing the expression of VDRs).

And as we shall discover in chapter 6, on pages 171–173, cortisol controls bile acid reabsorption (Rose et al., 2011). Therefore corticosteroids almost surely help to reduce diarrhea by improving bile acid reabsorption. So from this insight we might conclude that

1. Corticosteroids suppress mast cell numbers.
2. Maintaining a sufficient vitamin D level is important for controlling inflammation.
3. Corticosteroids may help to reduce diarrhea by improving bile acid reabsorption.

The reason why reducing mast cell numbers helps to control inflammation should be apparent in view of the fact that increasing mast cell populations tend to promote increased mast cell activity. This results in an increase in the number of mast cell degranulations that result in the inappropriate release of histamine and other proinflammatory agents. If a more detailed explanation of the complete process whereby the active form of vitamin D is capable of controlling mast cell numbers and activity level, and how corticosteroids work by exploiting the ability of vitamin D to control mast cell populations and activity, please see pages 55–69 of the book *Vitamin D and Autoimmune Disease* (Persky, 2014).[51]

Antihistamines can be used to help prevent the relapse of symptoms that usually occurs when a budesonide treatment regimen is ended.

Associated with this mast cell rebound issue, epidemiological evidence shows that taking an antihistamine daily when nearing the end of a budesonide treatment regimen and for a week or two afterward can help to maintain remission. This effect has not yet been documented in the medical literature, so this explanation is strictly opinion (not medically proven fact), but my opinion of why antihistamines are beneficial when ending a budesonide treatment is as follows:

In addition to histamine, cytokines, and other pro-inflammatory agents, mast cells also release serotonin when they degranulate. Antihistamines inhibit serotonin uptake. About 90 % of the serotonin in our bodies is located in our enterochromaffin (EC) cells in the epithelia of our intestines. Serotonin released from EC cells regulates motility in the gut (in the brain serotonin affects mood, and other attributes). One of the primary problems with any type of colitis is the regulation of intestinal motility.

As we just finished discussing, corticosteroids (including budesonide) primarily work by suppressing mast cell numbers and activity. Weaning off a corticosteroid typically results in a rebound of the number of mast cells and their activity level (greater numbers means increased activity), which tends to promote increased motility. Therefore, weaning too fast can cause mast cell numbers to rebound and overshoot their normal population and activity level, which can result in diarrhea in many cases. So in my opinion antihistamines help in this situation by utilizing the inhibition of serotonin uptake to suppress motility, which thereby limits the risk of increased motility (and diarrhea) when weaning off a corticosteroid.

Understanding Microscopic Colitis

In retrospect, it seems very likely that the failure of gastroenterology specialists to recognize the significance of mast cells in inflammatory bowel disease may be a primary reason why so little real progress has been made in the options available for treating MC and other IBDs during the past quarter century. Diagnosis of MC cases has increased significantly during this period of time due to the increased use of colonoscopy exams and especially due to the increased use of biopsies to identify the disease. But the types of medical treatments available have changed little during all those years.

The primary reason why this is so important is because the association of mast cell activity with MC suggests that many environmental factors can affect the disease. These can range from food or other dietary allergens to classic allergy issues such as seasonal pollen. Some patients even react to mild chemical vapors (such as cleaning agents), molds, and heat (even exercise-based heat increases).

Consider the fact that many MC patients complain that 10 to 20 minutes after they begin eating a meal, they have to run to the bathroom. According to the official medical understanding of the disease, this type of reaction cannot be explained. Conventional thinking says that the inflammation associated with MC is due to the infiltration of inflammation-promoting lymphocytes into the mucosal lining of the colon. But this is a relatively slow reaction, because it must first be initiated by the production of IgA antibodies as the immune system reacts to antigens in the diet, and then the IgA antibodies must subsequently promote the infiltration of additional lymphocytes and other pro-inflammatory mediators This typically results in approximately a 3–6-hour lag between the ingestion of food and an episode of secretory diarrhea (watery diarrhea).for most MC patients.

So how could it be possible that a reaction to a meal could trigger an episode of "explosive" diarrhea in as few as 10 to 20 minutes (or less)?

Only IgE-based reactions can proceed that quickly. Ige-based reactions primarily involve the degranulation of mast cells to release histamine and other pro-inflammatory agents. Obviously this type of reaction pattern would support the theory of the association of mast cell activity with MC symptoms.

Problems with gluten sensitivity first surfaced approximately 10,000 years ago as agriculture was developed and wheat was initially introduced into the diet of many early settlements as the neolithic period in human evolution began. Celiac disease was medically defined during the first century AD by a Greek physician named Aretaeus of Cappadocia, who wrote, "If the stomach be irretentive of the food and if it pass through undigested and crude, and nothing ascends into the body, we call such persons coeliacs" (Guandalini, 2007, summer. P. 1). But it took approximately 19 more centuries before a Dutch pediatrician happened to notice that when bread was rationed in the Netherlands during World War II, his patients' symptoms improved. And after the war, when bread became available again, their symptoms promptly became worse again. Working with other researchers, Dr. Dicke and his associates determined that gluten from wheat and rye was the cause of celiac disease.

In view of such slow progress in the medical understanding and recognition of the role that gluten sensitivity plays in celiac disease, it shouldn't be inappropriate to speculate that the failure to recognize the association of mast cells with MC might also very likely be a major part of the reason why most physicians still fail to recognize the role played by food sensitivities in the perpetuation of MC symptoms. We have to remember that up until relatively recently no researchers had ever published compelling medical research data based on random controlled trials to either verify or refute the claim that food sensitivities might be responsible for the chronic inflammation in many MC cases. But for some unknown reason, in the total absence of medical proof either pro or con, most clinicians have traditionally chosen to mistakenly assume that diet has nothing to do with the disease.

Interestingly, the well-known connection of the disease with drug-induced inflammation in many cases is not usually questioned by most physicians even though the effect has never been verified by rigid, random controlled research trials. The connection is always described as an "association" based on epidemiological evidence, but no one has ever published valid medical proof that the suspected drugs do indeed trigger the disease.

And yet most gastroenterologists readily understand that in cases of drug-induced MC, simply discontinuing the drugs that are suspected of causing the disease will sometimes bring remission, and the remission will typically remain in effect over the long term provided that the patient continues to avoid the class of drugs that triggered their disease. And additionally, many clinicians recognize that if a patient is using a medication known to trigger the disease, conventional medical treatments based on the use of anti-inflammatory medications will often fail to produce results unless the use of certain drugs known to trigger the disease are discontinued and avoided.

And yet many of these same physicians may routinely dismiss the suggestion that unresolved food sensitivities might be the cause of treatment failures. Why an obvious bias exists against the recognition of the possible role of inflammation caused by food sensitivities in the treatment of MC remains a mystery. This phenomenon can perhaps best be understood when we consider that physicians are trained to prescribe the use of drugs to treat symptoms, and they have virtually no training in the effects of food sensitivities on the digestive system. We will revisit the association of mast cells and MC in Chapter 5 to explore the relationship in more detail.

Incidentally, a very good ranking of drugs that may cause MC can be found in an article titled "Drug Exposure and the Risk of Microscopic Colitis: A Critical Update" (Lucendo, 2017).[52] This article rates drugs known or thought to cause MC by categories (high likelihood, intermediate likelihood, and low likelihood), so it's an excellent reference for anyone who has, or suspects they might have, drug-induced MC.

The full extent of the ways in which the digestive process is compromised when the intestines are inflamed is rather poorly understood.

It's likely that a large part of the problem is due to the loss of vital digestive enzymes as a direct result of the inflammation. If the surface area of the inner lining (the epithelia) of the small intestine were calculated, it would span a surprisingly large area. The internal surface area of the small intestine typically amounts to over 2,500 square feet (over232 square meters) By comparison, this is close to the size of a tennis court. That's a lot of surface area on which something can go wrong. And things definitely begin to go wrong when chronic inflammation becomes well established.

The disease is incorrectly named and incorrectly described.

As we learned in the first edition, despite the fact that collateral inflammation of the small intestine appears to be involved in most cases of MC (and this has been substantiated by numerous research articles that were referenced in the first edition), most medical professionals tend to treat the disease as though it were restricted to the colon because that's the way that the disease was originally incorrectly described in the medical literature. The word "Colitis" means inflammation of the colon.

But the inflammation is not restricted to the colon, and it's high time the medical profession corrected that mistake. Similar to Crohn's disease, many, many published medical research articles have shown that the pattern of inflammation associated with MC can adversely affect many other parts of the digestive system, and inflammation of the small intestine is a very common characteristic of MC (Koskela, 2011, Simondi et al., 2010, Wolber, Owen, & Freeman, 1990, Fine, Lee, & Meyer, 1998).[53, 54, 55, 56]

And if the evidence published in the medical literature is not sufficient, consider the fact that I, personally, had a colectomy in 2010 (because of a bleeding disorder that had nothing to do with MC). In other words, my colon was surgically removed. And yet if I slip up on my diet, I still experience most of the symptoms of microscopic colitis, so the disease is clearly still present. The removal of my colon made no significant difference in the status of the disease, as far as I can tell. Obviously, the evidence shows that the medical definition of the disease is incorrect. But will the medical description of the disease ever be corrected? Probably not any time soon.

Why do treatments by diet changes often fail?

Most dietary treatments fail because of lack of attention to detail or intentional deviations from a safe diet. We know this because of research that shows that at least a third of celiacs do not fully adhere to a gluten-free diet, despite the fact that their disease requires a gluten-free diet in order to treat their condition (Barratt, Leeds, & Sanders, 2011, Matoori, Fuhrmann, & Leroux, 2013).[57, 58] While a small amount of contamination of the diet may be due to accidental causes, apparently some celiacs believe that "a little bit won't hurt". Unfortunately a little bit does indeed negatively affect their health.

No studies of dietary compliance regarding MC patients have been published of course because dietary treatment of MC has not yet been recognized as an official medical treatment method for MC by the mainstream medical community. Nevertheless, surely similar dietary compliance problems occur with MC patients much as they do with celiac patients, due to both accidental and intentional diet contamination issues.

Of course not every failure is due to diet contamination. In many cases, the diet may not work correctly because it includes undiscovered food sensitivities. Or in some cases a combination of ingredients that are fine individually cause problems when combined. Problems of this nature may be very difficult to track down because when an ingredient is known to be generally safe, we naturally tend to assume it should be safe in all situations.

If we only include a single processed product in our diet and everything else is made from scratch, so that it's pure and free from gluten, then if there is any gluten in the processed product, it will be diluted by the other foods. Even if the gluten content happens to slightly exceed the legal limit of 20 parts per million, we will probably be safe, due to the dilution by other foods.

But if, for example, we choose to eat all processed foods, and each product contains the legal limit of 20 ppm, then everything we eat is pushing the legal limit for gluten and there's no dilution. If one of those products is mislabeled, and it accidentally contains more than the legal limit of gluten, we're probably in trouble. Or maybe we just happen to be someone who is more sensitive than normal, and we tend to react to anything that exceeds 10 ppm of gluten. Without the dilution by other safe foods, we will be more likely to react.

The point is, when gluten-free foods are allowed to have a legal built-in tolerance level, the total percentage of processed foods in our diet matters — the gluten is cumulative even though it's allowed on a percentage of total weight basis. We react based on the total amount of gluten consumed, rather than the percentage contained in an individual food. If we happen to use products or ingredients that all contain nearly the allowed legal limit of gluten, then the total amount of gluten consumed may be too much to tolerate for some individuals, while others might have no problem with it. This is just one of the reasons why patients who are following a recovery diet are more likely to reach remission, and reach it sooner, if they avoid all processed foods.

Health "experts" love to talk about "healthy" food, and "healthy" diets.

But no food can actually be healthy when it is eaten, because it is dead (or it soon will be). Food may have been healthy at one time (while it was still alive) but that time is past when it gets to someone's plate. So referring to it as healthy is incorrect. What we actually want is nutritious food, because if our food is nutritious, then we will be healthy, provided that our digestive system is capable of extracting and absorbing the nutrients contained on those foods.

Therein lies a primary problem because unfortunately most people who have MC or any other IBD tend to have compromised digestion when the disease is active. And some patients have compromised digestion to some extent at all times, due to permanent damage to various organs in the digestive system. When this is happening, it doesn't matter how nutritious the food might be, only a fraction of the nutrients that could normally be utilized (by a healthy digestive system) will actually be properly digested and absorbed. This may not be a problem in the short term, but if the malabsorption of nutrients goes on long enough, eventually deficiency problems will be very likely to develop, especially regarding certain vitamins and minerals.

And if the immune system produces antibodies to certain foods, resulting in an adverse reaction, then those foods can no longer be considered to be nutritious options. Instead, they must be viewed as toxic, because they do indeed impose a toxic threat to the body. Consequently they should no longer be thought of as "food", because they are no longer a safe food option.

Despite the fact that collagenous colitis was described over 4 decades ago, the disease is still poorly understood.

Part of the problem is that collagenous colitis was originally described in the medical literature as associated with frequent diarrhea, and because of that, many physicians still incorrectly believe the disease is only associated with diarrhea. Yet many cases involve alternating diarrhea and constipation or even constipation alone. This was finally documented in 2003 by Barta, Toth, Szabo, & Szegedi, and the original description of the disease was called into question.[59] But some medical professionals have never been able to get past the original description, and they still think of the disease as though it were only associated with diarrhea.

It's hardly surprising that physicians might have trouble understanding the disease. Much of what they are taught in medical school is misleading. A huge part of the problem can be found in the fact that like MC, celiac disease is incorrectly described. Physicians are taught that celiac disease is a disease of the small intestine. But that's simply not true. As previously discussed, celiac disease can (and frequently does) actually affect both the small and large bowel, and inflammation can be found in both when celiac disease is not properly treated.

And in many cases of celiac disease there are no significant clinical symptoms associated with the digestive system (at least not early on). Instead, the disease affects the brain and the central nervous system first. In some cases gastroenterological symptoms may never develop. Research shows that this is quite common (Hadjivassiliou et al., 1997, Hadjivassiliou, Grünewald, & Davies-Jones, 2002).[60, 61] But sadly, most physicians seem to be totally unaware of this huge group of celiac patients because of their inadequate training.

The obsolete tests currently used for diagnosing celiac disease are so insensitive that even the vast majority of celiacs who do have gastrointestinal symptoms are often not properly diagnosed. Some authorities are quick to point out that only about 1 in 20 celiacs are ever officially diagnosed. And one of the most perplexing and frustrating problems associated with that dilemma is the very unprofessional habit that many physicians seem to develop whereby they assume that any patient who has a negative result on a celiac screening test cannot be gluten sensitive. While it's true that a positive result on a celiac screening test is very good evidence of gluten sensitivity, no one has ever proven that a negative result rules out gluten sensitivity. So why would so many physicians make such a serious mistake? This has to link back to improper training. The truth is, in an unacceptably large percentage of cases, the classic celiac screening test is simply not sensitive enough to detect the disease; a fact that has been verified by medical research (Abrams, Diamond, Rotterdam, & Green, 2004).[62]

But beyond the problems with poor sensitivity of the blood tests used for screening for celiac disease, an even bigger disaster can be found in the upper endoscopy criteria considered to be the "gold standard" for a diagnosis of celiac disease. In order to confirm a diagnosis of celiac disease, biopsies taken from the small intestine of a patient must show total villus atrophy. In other words, the villi must be, for all practical purposes, totally flattened and no longer functional. Now why on earth would any physician need to wait until the villa of any patient's small intestine are totally dysfunctional? In practice, that degree of damage can take years to develop. Why must any patient be forced to suffer for so long in order to get a simple diagnosis? It should be sufficiently obvious that celiac disease is in progress long before the villi are totally destroyed.

It's unfortunate that unless a patient is willing to go through extensive suffering, they must look outside the medical community for help in order to get prompt resolution of symptoms. And woe be to anyone who dares to adopt a gluten-free diet without the blessing of the medical community. They will be ridiculed and scorned for trying to take care of their own health needs without an official celiac diagnosis.

Sometimes just plain poor digestion can prevent the remission of symptoms.

Whether caused by a deficiency of stomach acid, too much histamine, inflammation, or some other digestive problem, poor digestion can prolong the symptoms of MC. When we are unable to digest food normally, the partially-digested food tends to ferment in the warm, moist environment of our digestive system, resulting in the production of gas, bloating, and cramps. Obviously this cannot help the healing process and it may add to the total time needed for recovery.

The digestibility varies for different types of starch.

In general, overcooking cannot change the basic characteristics of any type of starch. Therefore while overcooking might possibly deplete some of the nutrients available (if the water is discarded after cooking the food), it shouldn't change the enzymes required for digestion after cooking. Starch characteristics are determined by the genetics of the plant, not by cooking. However, starch can be converted to sugar, and vice versa, by the proper enzymes. But again, this occurs independently of cooking. For example, when a seed-producing plant is growing, just prior to maturity the sugar in the endosperm of the seed is converted into starch, so that it will have a much better storage life. Then when a seed begins to germinate, an enzyme is released that progressively converts the starch in the endosperm back into sugar so that the developing sprout can easily use it as food. A similar process occurs in the human digestive system, when starch is degraded to sugars and further split by specific enzymes.

There are 2 basic types of starch, amylopectin and amylose.

Amylopectin is much easier to digest than amylose starch. Common starch is made of about 70% amylopectin by weight, though this fraction varies depending on the genetics of the plant that produces it. The rest is amylose. Higher amylopectin percentages are found in medium-grain rice (which can go up to 100% in glutinous rice), waxy potatoes, and waxy corn (maize), for example, so they are easier to digest.

Long-grain rice, amylomaize, and russet potatoes are examples of foods that contain lower fractions of amylopectin and higher percentages of amylose, so they are more difficult to digest. Waxy potatoes, which include red and yellow potatoes, for example, are much easier to digest than russet potatoes.

Amylose starch is sometimes referred to as "resistant starch" because of it's higher resistance to digestion, often resulting in incomplete digestion. Because of this characteristic, foods containing resistant starches (high amylose content) are often thought of as diet foods, implying that one can eat more of them while reducing the risk of gaining weight (because they are usually not completely digested). In my opinion this is a very poor way to go about dieting, since partially-digested or undigested foods are an open invitation to opportunistic bacteria that will ferment the residue in the colon, resulting in gas, bloating, and possibly diarrhea. At any rate, resistant starches should be avoided by anyone who is trying to recover from an MC flare

Actually,carbs are contraindicated not only for IBDs, but for human health in general.

The neolithic period in our history ushered in an unhealthy trend toward adding increasing amounts of carbohydrates to our diet. It's common knowledge that low-carb diets improve digestion and prevent heartburn, acid reflux, GERD, and various other digestive issues. Yet mostly due to the encouragement of various self-appointed "food police", we've added carbs to our diet until they dominate the diet.

As we've already discussed, the inflammation associated with IBDs results in a progressive loss of the ability to produce the digestive enzymes necessary to digest complex carbohydrates (complex sugars. This is one of the main reasons, along with the production of antibodies associated with certain proteins resulting from leaky gut, why digestion goes downhill, and malabsorption problems escalate, as MC develops.

This viewpoint (digestive difficulty) also suggests that fiber is contraindicated for MC. This is an issue with fiber that virtually everyone overlooks — fiber is a complex carbohydrate. In other words, like all carbs, when digested, the metabolites are sugars. Because fiber is a complex sugar (despite the fact that most people don't think of it that way), it tends to be difficult to digest. Of course this refers to digestible fibers (soluble fibers) — the insoluble fibers (such as cellulose) cannot be digested by the human digestive system, so they are fermented in the colon by bacteria.

This matters because sugars/carbs are totally unnecessary in the human diet.

Protein and fat are essential for good health, and also for our very survival, in the long run. Humans can not only totally do without carbs, but they tend to be healthier without them. This was proven to a skeptical medical community back in the 1930s, and then quickly forgotten by said medical community.[63]

When everything else fails, and ordinary elimination diets refuse to bring remission, an all-meat diet may provide a ticket to remission. It's definitely worth trying when nothing else seems to work.

Are probiotics helpful for treating MC?

The Microscopic Colitis Foundation insists that for most individuals, they are not helpful, and in a few cases they may even prevent some patients from being able to achieve remission.[64] And after years of claiming that probiotics were beneficial when included in an MC treatment program, even the American Gastroenterological Association Institute now agrees that in most cases, probiotics are not helpful when trying to bring an MC patient to remission and they specifically recommend against the use of probiotics when treating microscopic colitis.[65]

This intolerance of probiotic bacteria may be reflected in the fact that MC patients are likely to not be able to tolerate vegetables in the diet unless they are well-cooked. Raw vegetables are almost always poorly tolerated. While this is generally attributed to the inability to tolerate the irritating effects of fiber while the gut is inflamed, it may also be due to the bacteria found on and in many raw vegetables. Researchers have found that vegetables contain many more species of bacteria than we previously realized. For example, a single spinach leaf may contain more than 800 different species of bacteria.

In some cases, medications are a primary reason why a patient is unable to reach remission.

Be sure to consider all of the medications you are taking if you are in a flare and you can't find the cause. A few years ago many drugs were suspected of causing MC.

But now there are researchers who claim that after additional study, it appears that only nonsteroidal anti-inflammatory drugs (NSAIDS) and proton pump inhibitors (PPIs) cause MC (Masclee, Coloma, Kuipers, & Sturkenboom, 2015).[66] Nevertheless, the researchers concede that other drugs may make certain symptoms worse. In the absence of any published random, controlled trials, we can only make educated guesses.

Lactose in pharmaceutical products.

Theoretically, pure lactose in medications should not be a an issue because the only problem with lactose is that we cannot digest significant amounts of it when our gut is inflamed. Lactose is a sugar and sugars (with only one rare exception — alpha gal) do not cause the human immune system to produce antibodies. Only proteins can promote inflammation by triggering an immune system reaction. Casein is the dairy protein that is known to cause us to react (although we may also react to some of the proteins in whey).

Undigested sugars should simply pass through the small intestine unabsorbed into the colon. There they will usually be fermented by bacteria, causing some gas, but the small amounts (of sugars) in pills should be relatively insignificant so that fermentation of that small amount shouldn't cause any noticeable symptoms. At least that's the theory. If pharmaceutical companies use pharmaceutical grade lactose, then it should be pure, and pure lactose should contain no casein.

The problem is that in the real world many MC patients seem to react to lactose in at least some pharmaceutical products. This suggests the possibility that some pharmaceutical companies may be cheating and using cheaper industrial grade lactose rather than pharmaceutical grade lactose in some products. Industrial lactose contains traces of casein and whey because it is not as well purified as pharmaceutical grade lactose.

Many (possibly most) pharmaceutical ingredients are sourced from distant lands these days (China is a huge supplier, for example), and so if any cheating takes place, it probably occurs at the facilities of the suppliers of these ingredients (while the big pharmaceutical companies look the other way). But of course there is no proof to substantiate this suspicion. The bottom line is that probably some ingredients may be contaminated and some are not. If a product works OK for most patients, then there is a good chance that it may be pure.

Thyroid medication dosage may need to be adjusted during and after a corticosteroid treatment.

Corticosteroids suppress TSH, complicating thyroid treatments. This can cause hyperthyroid symptoms while being treated with a corticosteroid, and hypothyroid symptoms may return after a corticosteroid treatment is ended Therefore if you take a thyroid medication in order to correct a hypothyroid condition, expect your thyroid medication to be more potent while you are taking a corticosteroid. It may become necessary to lower the dose of your thyroid medication Your TSH should be back to normal after the corticosteroid treatment is over. If you are normally hyperthyroid instead, you may find it necessary to increase the dose of your thyroid medication while taking a corticosteroid and lower it again after the corticosteroid treatment is ended.

Of course if you have not adjusted your dose of whatever thyroid medication you are taking after starting the corticosteroid treatment, then it shouldn't be necessary to change the dose after the corticosteroid treatment regimen is ended. Normally, this only becomes a significant problem in cases where a patient is very hypothyroid and a corticosteroid is used for a relatively long period of time. It shouldn't be a factor for most patients.

Shared utensils are a common source of cross-contamination.

In some cases, utensils used for cooking and eating are a frustrating cause of cross-contamination, especially when someone in the household does not eat gluten free, so that the utensils are exposed to gluten regularly. In such cases the first incorrectly or incompletely done dish washing will result in cross-contamination. This problem can be very difficult to track down because it tends to be an assumed-safe part of the daily routine. Using dedicated utensils is the obvious solution because it eliminates the cross-contamination risk. Washing dishes, knives and forks, and pots and pans separately from gluten-contaminated utensils will help ensure that gluten-free utensils remain absolutely gluten free. Cross-contamination from utensils may only pose the risk of exposure to a tiny amount of gluten, but it adds up , and over time it can be a major problem that can easily prevent remission.

Why shouldn't everyone try a gluten free diet?

Adopting a gluten-free diet is obviously not something to be done as a whim — it's a major lifestyle change, a commitment that's likely to affect every part of the rest of your life. While it's probably true that everyone's long-term health would benefit if they avoided gluten, there's a caveat here to keep in mind. If we are predisposed to be sensitive to gluten, in other words, if we have the genes that predispose us to gluten sensitivity (and approximately 96 % of the general population do), in many cases, eliminating gluten from our diet will increase our immune system's sensitivity to it. Many people (probably most people) have developed some degree of sensitivity to gluten, but they have no clinical symptoms because they have been eating it all their life, and so their immune system has developed a tolerance for it. Once gluten has been eliminated from the diet for an extended period of time however, future exposures may trigger a reaction, even though it was it was well-tolerated before.

This may seem to be a paradox, but it's similar to oral immunotherapy treatments where allergists treat allergies by exposing the patient to tiny but increasing doses of an allergen until their immune system develops a tolerance to it so that a normal exposure does not trigger a reaction. However, the catch to this therapy is that the patient has to continue regular (preferably daily) exposures to the allergen, or she or he will lose tolerance and begin to react again. As long as they continue to ingest a maintenance dose of the allergen, they are fine, possibly for the rest of their life. But if they stop the maintenance therapy, they are likely to lose their tolerance. Many people have induced tolerance to gluten, so a decision to eliminate it from the diet may become a permanent necessity, by default. So gluten-free is not only a way of life, but an irreversible choice, in most cases.

What are the risks of cheating on one's diet?

If you're ever inclined to take a chance and cheat on your restricted diet, cheating with gluten is not a good choice because the half-life of anti-gliadin (anti-gluten) antibodies is 120 days. That means that a few minutes of indiscretion can result in months of increased inflammation. The half-life of most other food antibodies, by comparison, is only about

6 days. And cheating on fiber has the least amount of extended influence. Eating too much fiber may result in an adverse reaction, but fiber does not provoke the immune system to produce any antibodies, so it's less likely to cause a major setback.

It's natural to want to experiment by reintroducing foods. Unfortunately it takes a lot longer for the gut to heal than almost everyone realizes — typically 2 to 3 years for most adults, and some cases take longer. Kids heal much faster — usually in less than a year. But because of the long half-life of anti-gliadin antibodies, they tend to dominate the immune system as long as the level is relatively high. As that level declines, then the immune system is once again able to focus on other antigens. Until our immune system recovers somewhat from the overpowering effects of gluten, it may be almost impossible to make sense of reaction symptoms.

The main problem with trying to reintroduce foods too soon (besides the inconvenience of a possible reaction) is that every failure bumps the inflammation level up a bit, which extends the recovery time. There is a good chance that the reason why daring to reintroduce a food and not having an adverse reaction has such a gratifying effect is because it not only proves that eating that food may be safe, but it has a very calming effect on stress levels. Stress promotes inflammation, and the absence of stress helps to resolve inflammation.

Why are stool tests much more reliable and accurate than blood or skin tests for detecting food sensitivities?

Allergists usually order blood tests that are designed to detect IgE (and maybe IgG) antibodies in the blood. If she or he does any skin tests those will likely be IgE tests. As mentioned on page 3 of this chapter, IgE tests are used to detect classic allergic reactions. These are mast cell reactions where histamines and other proinflammatory mediators are released to cause itching, swelling, redness, rash or hives, and other classic symptoms of an allergic reaction. In severe cases, IgE antibodies are also the ones that can cause life-threatening anaphylactic reactions where blood pressure may drop and it may become difficult to breathe because of airway constrictions. IgG antibodies are simply markers of chronic IgE-based reactions. The skin tests are mostly useful for skin allergies, and have little value for most MC Patients.

While many of us also have IgE antibody issues, these are not the cause of the intestinal inflammation associated with MC. The mechanism described in the medical literature as the classic cause of MC is T-cell promoted inflammation. T-cell activation can have many causes when the disease is initially triggered. But as the symptoms become chronic, this mode of inflammation is perpetuated by antibodies produced in response to food sensitivities within the digestive system. The proliferation of T-cell infiltration into the mucosal lining of the intestines is in response to IgA antibodies produced by the immune system in response to food sensitivities.

Because of the lack of training in this area in med school, most allergists are not usually concerned with IgA antibodies, so they aren't even aware of the fact that IgA antibodies promote intestinal inflammation. They mostly understand IgE and IgG antibodies, because of their training and experience. As a result, their testing methods are usually not particularly relevant to the food sensitivities that are associated with MC, though occasionally some of the foods that show positive test results in the blood or skin tests will also show positive results when tested for IgA antibodies (in stool). But even if allergists tested for IgA antibodies (in blood), the antibodies are produced in the gut, not in the blood, so the blood level of IgA antibodies caused by food sensitivities is typically so low that the blood tests are very unreliable for detecting antibodies caused by food sensitivities in the gut. And the skin tests are even less appropriate for detecting food sensitivities.

For example, it often takes years for the antibody level to build up in the blood to a sufficient level where it is likely to yield a positive celiac test result (based on IgA and IgG antibodies) in celiacs. By that time the patient has typically suffered from clinical symptoms for many months or years, and their intestine has accrued severe damage. But a stool test will detect the antibodies even before clinical symptoms appear. IOW, the stool tests are several orders of magnitude more sensitive, and they will detect celiac disease several years sooner (in most cases) than the classic celiac blood tests. Currently, accurate and reliable food sensitivity testing (stool testing) is only available on the Internet, from Entero-Lab.

Why doesn't the calprotectin test reliably detect the inflammation associated with MC?

While the calprotectin test is useful for detecting the inflammation associated with Crohn's disease and UC, it rarely shows an elevated test result for microscopic colitis. Why does that happen? It happens because the calprotectin test result indicates significant migration of neutrophils into the intestinal mucosa. Significant neutrophil infiltration does not normally occur with MC, though neutrophils are indeed significantly involved with the inflammation pattern associated with Crohn's disease and UC. So a negative result on a calprotectin test rules out Crohn's disease and ulcerative colitis, but does not rule out microscopic colitis.

Summary

In chapter one we discussed many possibilities that can contribute to or cause a treatment program to fail. A single problem can cause a treatment failure., or the lack of success can be due to a combination of issues. But the main thing to remember is that in tough cases, every sensitivity issue may need to be addressed. In the easy cases, remission comes easily and minor problems can sometimes be ignored. While in other cases, virtually everything may need to be addressed in order to gain complete control over the symptoms.

Chapter 2

Cross-Contamination and Other Dietary Issues

If diet changes don't help, cross-contamination or unrecognized sensitivities are common reasons for treatment failure.

Many MC patients are unable to achieve remission, and yet when questioned about the possibility of cross-contamination of their diet by gluten they typically respond with something like, "But I'm extremely careful — I don't see how my diet could be cross-contaminated with gluten." Believe me, it can be cross-contaminated, despite the fact that you are being extremely careful. Gluten is so ubiquitous that it can sneak in under our radar to contaminate our diet. It's sometimes where we least expect it to be, right under our nose. But sometimes we make it easy for gluten to sneak in.

Is there a bag of wheat flour in your house?

Is someone in your household not gluten-free? If there' a bag of wheat flour in your home, your diet is going to be cross-contaminated. The risk is so high as to be virtually a sure thing in my opinion.

Understanding Microscopic Colitis

To see the risk, open a bag of flour early or late in the day when the sun is low and streaks of sunlight are streaming in through a window. The number of particles that can be seen drifting around in all directions in those light beams will surprise you. Or just drop an unopened bag of flour a couple of inches onto a countertop and look at all the flour that gets blown into the air, even though the bag hasn't yet been opened. Wheat flour is so fine that it billows up and goes everywhere. And it settles on everything — not only on tables and countertops and every-thing else that's exposed, but smaller amounts also settle on dishes and utensils stored in cabinets and drawers. And every time a cabinet door is opened, air currents sweep some flour particles into the air. Every time someone walks through the room, flour particles billow up from the slight air currents caused by the movement. Wheat flour is insidious stuff. Any celiac living within several hundred yards of a flour mill would surely always show relatively high anti-gliadin antibody levels, regardless of the direction of the prevailing winds, simply because the flour dust goes everywhere, and it never completely leaves — it just tends to be continually relocated by air currents. Yes, it can be wiped off countertops to remove a lot of it, but it can't be wiped out of the air, without sophisticated filtration systems.

Contamination from processed foods that contain gluten is relatively easy to avoid, because that gluten stays put. You just have to wipe up the crumbs and keep them off your food, wash your hands, and any-thing that might come into contact with your food. But wheat flour doesn't stay put. It's always on the move, looking for another place to hide, and another plate of food to contaminate. Celiacs who have rela-tively high tolerance levels may be able to tolerate wheat flour in the house if good cleanup practices are followed, but many individuals are too sensitive to tolerate those trace amounts, despite the best of precau-tions. And that applies to MC patients as well.

Reactions against gluten are due to an ancient immune system response that developed during our evolution.

Certain pathogens such as the bacteria that cause cholera (vibrio cholerae) cause increased intestinal permeability (aka leaky gut), so it's not surprising that our immune system would respond to an infection of that type. Interestingly, cholera causes the same type of watery diarrhea (secretory diarrhea) as MC. The rapid dehydration and the subsequent high risk of death that it causes is why cholera developed a reputation as such a dreaded disease. Yet microscopic colitis is rated as a benign disease by the medical community. Of course it's rarely fatal, but occasionally it can cause sometimes-fatal symptoms, such as dehydration.

At any rate, wheat unfortunately causes some of the same types of symptoms in our gut as cholera, that is, it increases intestinal permeability, which leads to secretory diarrhea. And it increases intestinal permeability not just for celiacs, but for everyone. Dr. Fasano and his crew of researchers at the University of Maryland Medical School proved that over 10 years ago (Drago et al., 2006). The intestinal permeability just increases faster for celiacs.

This happens every time someone eats gluten, and over time it takes its toll and the tight junctions open wider and wider as time goes on. Celiacs of course, and those who have at least one of the two main celiac genes, have a much more pronounced response than non-celiacs, so that they tend to reach the point at which leaky gut begins to allow peptides from partially-digested food to enter the bloodstream much sooner than non-celiacs. Once those peptides begin to enter the bloodstream, the immune system responses begin to become a major problem.

So yes, leaky gut triggers immune system responses that were designed to fight pathogens that cause increased intestinal permeability (such as cholera). Food was never intended to trigger that response because food never triggered increased intestinal permeability before gluten entered the human diet. And no food in the human diet could elicit that response until wheat was developed during the neolithic period of our history. Now that wheat has become ingrained in the human diet, everyone's immune system has become unnecessarily edgy and prone to react when it shouldn't, because we're eating a food that mimics one of the pathogenic actions of the cholera bacterium.

Consider the history of gluten sensitivity and celiac disease.

As was mentioned in chapter 1, gluten sensitivity, in the form of celiac disease, was first described in the medical literature approximately 2,000 years ago (Guandalini, 2007, summer. p. 1). But not much medical progress was made until the 1930s when Willem Dicke began a series of experiments using wheat-free diets, after reading the reports of a child who experienced diarrhea after eating bread or biscuits (Peña & Rodrigo, 2015).[67] He published his results in 1947 and presented them at the International Congress of Pediatrics. But his work was not taken seriously. So with the help of some colleagues, he showed that when wheat was removed from the diet of celiac patients, fecal fat was reduced. And reintroducing it resulted in a resumption of excess fat in the stool, a condition called steatorrhea, known to be associated with celiac disease.

These new data were presented at the International Congress of the International Pediatric Association in Zurich in 1950 and published in Acta Paediatrica Scandinavica (Dicke, Weijrs, & Van De Kamer, 1953).[68] Due to the rejection of the article by a prominent American publication, its final publication was delayed. Apparently there was publication bias against medical articles that contradicted the popular view even in the 1950s. Concurrently, another group of researchers showed that the steatorrhea was due to a corruption of the process of intestinal absorption (Anderson et al., 1954).[69] So finally after about 2,000 years some progress was made in understanding celiac disease. But despite recent progress, much remains to be done regarding the medical understanding of gluten sensitivity.

Research shows that there are over 300 reactive peptides in various protein molecules of wheat, rye, and barley. Ever wonder why there are so many? It turns out that wheat was arguably the worst possible grain choice for the designation of "staff-of-life". The evidence is in the wheat genome – it contains so many more opportunities for proteins that can trigger reactions. Wheat has several orders of magnitude more genes than any other grain. In fact, wheat has somewhere between roughly 8 and 15 times as many genes as humans. With such a huge number of genes, the statistical odds of corruption go way up. So it's no wonder that there are so many peptide possibilities that cause so many people to react.

Occasionally mislabeling is the cause of diet cross-contamination.

In some cases a cross-contaminated diet is the result of an oversight, an incorrect assumption, lack of information, or some other reason that causes a product to be mislabeled. Sometimes manufacturers change ingredients, and this type of label change can easily be overlooked It's human nature to assume that a food product that was safe the last time we purchased it should be safe the next time we purchase it. But unfortunately that isn't always the case, and quite often, label changes on products or mislabeled products will show up on food store shelves. Whether the mistake is due to lack of coordination between ingredient changes and labeling changes, or a communication failure between an ingredient supplier and the product manufacturer, the effect on the consumer is the same — an unanticipated adverse reaction, if the consumer happens to be sensitive to an ingredient that is omitted from, or incorrectly represented on the label.

Some food ingredients are not safe for MC patients despite "expert" claims to the contrary.

One of the most insidious label problems is the case where a mistake is made based on an incorrect "expert" opinion. For example, most industry "experts" agree that soy oil and soy lecithin do not contain any soya protein, and therefore they are safe for anyone who is sensitive to soy. Unfortunately that opinion is based on a misunderstanding of the facts, and the real-world experiences of many individuals who are sensitive to soy show that while soy lecithin may be safe for some, soy oil may be a problem for most.

Process engineers design and develop such separation processes, and any process engineer is well aware that perfect processes exist only in theory. In the real world, all mechanical and chemical separation processes are imperfect, and every last one of them results in a certain percentage of residues that are typically ignored, because they are simply written off as "within the allowed tolerances" for the process. And so non-engineering "experts" are naive enough to believe that as long as tolerance limits are maintained, the process results in "pure" products.

But of course the products are not actually pure. Those small contamination levels that fall within the specified tolerance limits of the process may seem so tiny as to be irrelevant, but they are not irrelevant to many immune systems, where minuscule amounts may be sufficient to trigger a reaction in many cases.

Tolerances are usually specified in thousandths or ten thousandths, whereas sensitivities are usually specified in parts per million (ppm). A thousandth is a thousand times as large as a ppm, and a ten thousandth is a hundred times as large as a ppm. So the tolerance allowances used for the processes are far too great (many orders of magnitude) to guarantee purity for anyone who is sensitive to these proteins. In the case of soy lecithin, the processing usually neutralizes the protein in the finished product so that it becomes harmless. But that's not the case with soy oils. The bottom line is that despite expert claims to the contrary, most products that contain soy oil are not safe for MC patients who are sensitive to soy. And as discussed in detail in the first edition of *Microscopic Colitis*, that caveat also applies to products used on the skin, or hair and scalp, again, despite "expert" claims to the contrary.

And in many cross-contamination situations, an unexpected complication comes into play. Recent research based on warnings about food safety involving toxins in certain foods suggests that most people tend to modify their perceptions of warnings about food risks if the information conflicts with their personal beliefs or personal preferences (Cornell Food & Brand Lab, 2015, November 24).[70] The net effect is that if a favorite food is involved, then for most people, the perceived risk is viewed as significantly lower than the actual risk. Some people will even totally ignore a warning if it conflicts with their beliefs. The implication is that information about risks is not sufficient to convince some or possibly most people to change their attitude, let alone convince them to change their behavior.

So clearly, if food safety warnings about possible toxins in food are not sufficient to change behavior among the general population, then it's no wonder that warnings about personal food sensitivities are not always recognized to be as important as they should be. And of course the risk with treatments based on diet changes is that a lower perception of risk, or a lower opinion of the importance of a recommendation can lead to less attention to details that may result in failure of the treatment to bring remission.

Certain loopholes in labeling laws may cause problems for those who have food sensitivities.

For example, many people are sensitive to sulfites. Sulfites are not one of the allergens required by law to be specifically listed as an allergen on labels. In fact, trace amounts of sulfites are exempt from even being mentioned on labels, according to U.S. Law. In the U. S., trace amounts are not defined by the regulations, so what are food manufacturers and processors to do? Generally, when an ingredient is present in what the FDA refers to as "incidental" amounts, and it has no functional or technical effect on the finished product, then it does not need to be listed on the label.

An incidental ingredient is usually present because it is normally found in another ingredient. This convention does not exempt the eight major food allergens (even if they are present in trace amounts — they must be specifically listed on the label under all circumstances. Sulfites that have been added to any food or any ingredient are considered to be an incidental level if they comprise 10 ppm or less of the finished product.[71] This is a relatively tight limit. But naturally-occurring sulfites appear to be exempt from this requirement.

Beware of natural flavors.

The term "natural flavors" amounts to a loophole in the current ingredient labeling laws. "Natural flavors" may sound safe, but a natural flavor is seldom actually "natural". In reality, natural flavors are typically highly processed chemicals which, by themselves or in combination with other chemicals, add a flavor to food. They're allowed to be called "natural" because the original source of the chemical additive is not man-made.

The FDA says (CFR - Title 21 2016, September 9):[72]

The term *natural flavor* or *natural flavoring* means the essential oil, oleoresin, essence or extractive, protein hydrolysate, distillate, or any product of roasting, heating or enzymolysis, which contains the flavoring constituents derived from a spice, fruit or fruit juice, vegetable or vegetable juice, edible yeast, herb, bark, bud, root, leaf or similar plant material, meat, seafood, poultry, eggs, dairy products, or fermentation products thereof, whose significant function in food is flavoring rather than nutritional. [Sec. 501.22, Item (3)]

Note that because food manufacturers are not required to disclose the ingredients of any "natural flavors" added, it can pretty much include anything, even something to which you may be severely allergic or intolerant. Also please be aware that any foods served in a restaurant may also contain "natural flavors," which will almost surely not be listed on the menu.

Fructose can be a problem for some MC patients, even in vegetables.

Some authorities claim that roughly 30 % of the general population have problems absorbing fructose. Similar to the digestive problems caused by lactose intolerance, unabsorbed fructose will pass into the colon, where it will be fermented by bacteria. This can result in gas, bloating, cramps, and diarrhea. Heat degrades fructose faster than other sugars, so making sure that vegetables are well-cooked helps to minimize or at least reduce fructose-intolerance problems. Vegetables that contain significant (but not large) amounts of fructose include asparagus, beans, broccoli, cauliflower, celery, cucumber, and leafy greens. The highest amounts of fructose are found in corn, carrots, sweet potatoes, and tomatoes. Technically, tomato is a fruit, not a vegetable, and of course when mature, corn is a cereal grain, not a vegetable.

Vegetables in the low-fructose category are safest for people who are fructose-intolerant. Vegetables in this category that seem to have the lowest risk of causing problems for MC patients include Brussels sprouts, beetroot, green beans, potatoes, squash, and zucchini. When over-cooked, asparagus, broccoli, cauliflower, celery, carrots, and sweet potatoes are also suitable for most people.

Note that most people who are fructose-intolerant do not necessarily have to totally avoid fructose. And that's fortunate, because totally avoiding fructose would be quite a challenge. They just have to limit their total intake of fructose so that the total amount in their system at all times remains below their personal threshold (tolerance level) at which it may begin to trigger symptoms. Obviously that's more easily done if foods with the highest amounts of fructose are avoided, or at least minimized in the diet.

The problem with vitamin E.

Vitamin E can be found listed on labels in various forms, including d-alpha tocopherol, dl-tocopherol, alpha tocopherol acetate, mixed tocotrienols, tocopheryl acetate, and vitamin E succinate. Most of these (other than the first two) are very ambiguous terms. The topic of the safety of vitamin E for anyone who is sensitive to soy comes up often.

Natural vitamin E (in food) occurs in eight different chemical forms, called isomers:

> alpha tocopherol
> beta tocopherol
> delta tocopherol
> gamma tocopherol
> alpha tocotrienol
> beta tocotrienol

76

delta tocotrienol
gamma tocotrienol

Note that the first 4 are tocopherols, while the other 4 are tocotrienols. It was initially thought that only alpha tocopherol is needed for human nutrition. So supplements that contain natural vitamin E typically only contain alpha tocopherol, and this is designated on labels as d-alpha-tocopherol. Unfortunately most of those supplements are derived from soy oil because of its relatively low price.

But about 99 % of the vitamin E supplements that are available, use synthetic alpha-tocopherol, designated as dl-alpha-tocopherol. Research shows that most synthetic vitamin E supplements are very poorly absorbed, so most health advocates shy away from synthetic vitamin E supplements. Synthetic forms of vitamin E are only about half as effective as natural forms of vitamin E. And unfortunately, virtually all vitamin E supplements (whether natural or synthetic) contain only a single isomer of vitamin E (based on alpha tocopherol).

But research shows that gamma tocopherol is actually the most common isomer found in food. In fact, roughly 70 % of the vitamin E found naturally in food is in the form of gamma tocopherol. That predominance in itself suggests that totally ignoring this isomer in vitamin E supplements is probably counterproductive. It's certainly counterintuitive at the very least. Why is this important? Because when only alpha tocopherol is supplemented, this tends to significantly deplete gamma tocopherol levels in the body because gamma tocopherol is needed by the body in order to reduce inflammation and regulate certain factors that protect against certain diseases (including certain cancers) (Moyad, Brumfield, &Pienta, 1999, Jiang, Christen, Shigenaga, & Ames, 2001).[73,74] Gamma tocopherol is also known to activate genes that protect against Alzheimer's disease.

So clearly, virtually all vitamin E supplements (whether natural or synthetic) are contraindicated for the prevention of certain diseases, including cancer and Alzheimer's, simply because they exclude gamma tocopherol, and because of that shortcoming, they tend to deplete existing supplies of gamma tocopherol in the body. The obvious goal should be to try to get vitamin E from food, not from supplements, and not from processed foods that are enriched with vitamin E in the form of various tocopherols.

Vitamin E is available in various foods, including almonds, sunflower seeds and oil, safflower oil, olive oil, spinach and other dark green leafy vegetables, broccoli, squash, shellfish, many fish, avocados, and certain fruits and berries. Most people who have MC can tolerate many of those foods, so it shouldn't be necessary to use any vitamin E supplements. And of course vitamin E is also available in peanuts and soybean oil, and in tomatoes, but most of us find it necessary to avoid those foods.

But most people who have MC are not concerned so much with getting enough vitamin E from food — they're much more concerned about accidentally ingesting a form of tocopherol derived from soy. As far as processed foods in general are concerned, far too many of them are "enriched" with some form of vitamin E, and the trick is to figure out which form of vitamin E is used, to determine whether or not it's safe to use. A "Soy-Free" banner on the label of the product cannot be relied upon, because most label designers do not recognize natural forms of tocopherols as a derivative of soy.

When natural forms of vitamin E are used (d-tocopherol), unless the source of the ingredient is otherwise specified, it's safest and usually most accurate to assume that the source is soy (because that's what it's usually made from). When the type of vitamin E is listed on the label as dl-alpha-tocopherol, or as synthetic vitamin E, then it does not contain any soy derivatives.

Any ingredient "extracts" should also be viewed with suspicion because in many cases the extraction medium used is soy oil. A good example of this is the rosemary extract found in most processed turkeys these days. Pure rosemary should be safe for most people who have MC, but rosemary extract may cause problems for anyone who is sensitive to soy.

Eating at restaurants can be quite a challenge.

The problem is that there is only one basic way that food preparation can go right, and thousands (or maybe tens of thousands) of ways that it can go wrong. And at the root of the problem is the fact that there is no way that most people who do not have the disease can comprehend the extent of the attention to detail that is required to successfully keep food safe. And that applies to each and every serving of food that is included in the meal. So the mathematical odds of receiving a complete meal that's actually safe (and not cross-contaminated), at a restaurant, would have to be incredibly slim.

What about digestive enzymes that are claimed to allow the digestion of gluten and casein?

Some of these products are promoted as though they will allow the user to ignore food sensitivities and eat previously forbidden foods. Unfortunately, similar to the situation with soy oil and soy lecithin, these enzymes do not allow perfect digestion processes. Some of the gluten-associated peptides and casein-associated peptides that cause reactions for MC patients are bound to get by without being split. And even though this may amount to only a very low percentage, it will typically be sufficient to cause most MC patients to react if enough gluten or casein is consumed.

And even if the number of undigested peptides is below the personal threshold at which a reaction will be triggered, there is a very good chance that the quantity will be more than adequate to maintain a state of chronic low-level inflammation in the body if the practice of using a digestive aid to justify the consumption of food sensitivities becomes routine. It's well known that even low-level chronic inflammation is very undesirable due to the increased risk of the development of autoimmune diseases. Therefore using these products as a workaround for food sensitivities would be a very impractical option. Doing so would surely jeopardize long-term health.

However, products such as these may be useful as sort of a "safety net" in situations where a risk of cross-contamination exists, such as when eating at restaurants or other locations away from home where trace amounts of gluten or casein might be encountered because dedicated facilities (or proper training) are not available for the preparation of gluten-free or casein-free food. Although such products should presumably work better if taken before such a meal, even if they are taken reasonably soon after a meal they may help to prevent, or at least reduce the severity of a reaction in situations where it is suspected that gluten or casein may have been unintentionally ingested.

Why is it so important to minimize fiber in the diet?

Fiber is traditionally considered a necessary part of the human diet. It's thought to improve motility. And indeed, for many people it will work as claimed. But one of the last things needed by most MC patients is increased motility. They need less motility, not more.

As Dr. Michael Eades points out in his blog, fiber works to "promote regularity" (as fiber fans love to claim) by irritating the cells of the mucosal lining of the gut (Eades, 2006, August 30). Fiber actually physically tears these cells and when that happens the immune system marks those cells for destruction and replacement, because it is easier to replace them than to try to repair them (Miyake, Tanaka, & McNeil, 2006, Underwood, 2006).[75, 76] Once the cell is marked for destruction (a process known as apoptosis), it dumps all of its mucin supply immediately. When combined with water, mucin makes mucus, which helps to lubricate the inside of the intestines, and this speeds up motility to help induce a bowel movement. And this thrills fiber fans because it prevents them from having to track down the problem with their diet that is causing constipation in the first place. I would point out that there are two very common causes of constipation and these causes are especially likely for most MC patients — dehydration and chronic magnesium deficiency. Most people who have MC tend to be prone to having both these problems.

The main point here is that the last thing most MC patients need is faster motility and another bowel movement, and they certainly don't need any additional damage to their intestines. Most MC patients have more than enough intestinal damage already, so the recommendations of physicians who advise MC patients to take fiber supplements are clearly counterproductive.

The safest policy regarding baked goods is to avoid all of them during recovery.

Random testing of gluten-free flours on store shelves shows that cross-contamination of these flours with gluten is somewhat common (Thompson, Lee, & Grace, 2010).[77] In some instances the amount of gluten contamination is only slightly above the maximum limit allowed by FDA regulations. But in other cases the amount is much more significant and could be enough to cause some individuals to react if they are sensitive to gluten.

Understanding Microscopic Colitis

In addition, some patients tend to react to certain combinations of flours, even though the individual flours might not cause any problems. Since gluten-free flours usually work better in combinations, rather than as individual flours, combining types of GF flours almost always improves the baking and texture characteristics of the finished product. But of course combining ingredients increases the odds of introducing contamination into the mix. The greater the number of ingredients, the higher the odds that the finished product may be cross-contaminated with gluten.

During a flare (and also during the initial recovery phase) the immune system is extremely sensitive, and it will tend to react to low levels of antigens that would probably be below the threshold necessary to trigger a reaction after stable remission has been in place for a few months or longer. Therefore it's necessary to use extra care to avoid even tiny trace amounts of foods known or suspected to be a problem, during the recovery phase. Anything that can be done to expedite recover or shorten the recovery time is usually well worth the extra effort.

Because of that risk, it's usually a good idea to avoid baked goods during the recovery period. Once stable remission has been achieved and a reasonable amount of time has passed to allow a significant amount of intestinal healing, baked goods can be tried experimentally to see if they might be safely added to the diet. But remember that every lot of flour may be different.

This is a much safer procedure than allowing baked goods in the diet during recovery, because any source of cross-contamination in the diet can prevent remission. And in that type of situation, there's typically no way of knowing exactly what caused the diet treatment to fail. A reaction to a specific food can only be reliably detected when stable remission is in place. If a reaction is already ongoing, there is no way to tell if a particular food is causing a reaction, or if the symptoms are simply part of the current flare.

Is it OK to drink coffee?

Most physicians recommend that coffee should be avoided by MC patients. Real world experience shows that most MC patients discover that if coffee sent them straight to the bathroom before their MC symptoms began, then it is very likely to do the same after MC develops. But on the other hand, if coffee did not initiate a prompt trip to the bathroom prior to the development of the disease, then it probably will not cause problems after MC develops. The biggest risk with coffee appears to be products that are added to the coffee rather than the coffee itself. Note that despite the fact that many coffee creamers are labeled as "Non-Dairy", they contain the ingredient "sodium caseinate" or some variation of that name. Sodium caseinate is the biochemical name for casein, which of course is the very ingredient in all dairy products that typically causes the immune system of many MC patients to produce antibodies.

Therefore, some MC patients drink their coffee black, some use almond milk, a few use coconut milk, or some other cow's milk alternative, and some use a small amount of cane sugar or sugar cubes. It's best to avoid artificial sweeteners such as aspartame because virtually everyone who has MC seems to have problems with most artificial sweeteners, especially during the recovery period, and experience shows that aspartame seems to be the worst of the available options. Some people claim that sucralose (Splenda) may be safer because it is derived from sugar, but unfortunately all artificial sweeteners affect gut bacteria populations. Gut bacteria population disruptions are already a problem for most MC patients, so additional problems in this area are not likely to be beneficial.

Is ghee a safe substitute for butter for those who are sensitive to casein?

Many people who are casein-sensitive naturally look at ghee, clarified butter, thinking it's free of casein. But the problem is that the way it's supposedly turned into a casein-free product is by a process that is often not reliable. Making ghee involves starting with ordinary butter and heating it to melt the butter so that the liquid separates from the milk solids which precipitate out and settle to the bottom of the container as globs of casein. The liquid (ghee) is then poured off or the globs of casein are simply filtered out to remove the casein. In essence, it's a simple process, but in reality it's fraught with peril. There's a substantial risk that the separation won't be complete, and if it isn't, the end product will be contaminated with casein.

If you do a little research based on the comments posted on many of the "thank goodness for ghee" blogs or forums you'll discover that many, many people do indeed react to ghee. And when they post that fact, someone will inevitably recommend a different brand. But that's not the solution. The sensible course of action is to simply stay away from ghee, because it's basically risky at best for anyone who is casein-sensitive. It was originally designed for gourmets, not patients with food sensitivities. This is especially important for people who have one or more autoimmune diseases, because like gluten, casein can sometimes cause very subtle symptoms for people who are sensitive to it. It often causes issues such as osteoarthritis, but the reaction is so slow that the connection is often overlooked.

Very pure ghee is 99.0 to 99.5 % pure. The best commercial ghee products fall into this category. But that leaves 0.5 to 1.0 % contamination, and 1.0 % (0.01) is 10,000 ppm — a massive amount, as food contaminants go. Using ghee is a bit like a celiac eating low-gluten bread — definitely not a good practice. And there's no telling what else might be in that 0.5 to 1.0 %.

Cross-reactivity may be a problem for some people.

The American Academy of Allergy, Asthma, & Immunology defines cross-reactivity thusly, "Cross-reactivity in allergic reactions occurs when the proteins in one substance (typically pollen) are similar to the proteins found in another substance (typically a food) (The American Academy of Allergy, Asthma & Immunology)."[78] Cross-reactivity can lead to food reactions according to certain patterns. For example, if one is allergic to birch pollen, then one may also react to apples, carrots, celery, hazelnuts, peaches, pears, and raw potatoes (Mayo Clinic staff, 2017).[79] In a similar fashion, ragweed pollen sensitivity can make one also react to bananas and melons, such as cantaloupe, honeydew, and watermelon. An allergy to grass pollen can also make one sensitive to melons, oranges, peanuts,tomatoes, and white potato. And an allergy to mugwort pollen can cause cross-reactivity with apples, bell peppers, carrots, celery, garlic, onion, and certain spices such as caraway seeds, parsley, coriander, anise seeds, and fennel seeds.

According to Dr. Amy Myers, at least six foods are capable of cross-reacting with gluten (Myers, n.d.).[80]

- Corn
- Dairy products such as milk and cheese (alpha-casein, beta-casein, casomorphin, butyrophilin, whey protein)
- Millet
- Oats
- Rice

- Yeast

Are food intolerances and allergies permanent?

For many years, specialists have been claiming that many children "outgrow" their childhood food intolerances. But the problem is that most do not actually outgrow them (Palmer, 2014, April 14).[81] It appears that chemical changes in the body, possibly associated with viruses or maybe with the hormonal changes that occur during adolescence, may be responsible for suppressing the symptoms of childhood allergies during adolescence and early adulthood, in some cases.

However, this theory has not been investigated, so it has not been proven by medical research. But medical statistics show that when those individuals reach their late 20s or early 30s, the symptoms often return. Sometimes they return as different symptoms.

For example, it is known that some children who outgrow a food allergy will later develop symptoms of eosinophilic esophagitis to that same food (Smith, 2014, March 18).[82] So the food intolerance obviously remains, even though the clinical symptoms may be different. This suggests that once someone's immune system begins to react to a food, that intolerance will probably last for the rest of that person's life, regardless of whether or not they always have clinical symptoms after eating the food.

As more research is done in the future, other immune system disorders that occur later in life will probably be discovered to be associated with childhood food intolerances that have been thought to be "outgrown". More and more medical professionals are realizing that inflammation, even when it is hidden, is the cause of all disease. That means that anything that can be done to minimize inflammation at all times may prevent the development of disease in the future. The simplest and safest way to prevent these problems from developing is to avoid those foods and never add them back into the diet.

When selecting olive oil, extra-virgin olive oil is the safest type for anyone with food sensitivities to use.

This is due to the ways that olive oil is processed. Extra-virgin olive oil is extracted by simply crushing the olives. Other types of olive oil may be extracted by a process that involves the use of chemicals. There are no clues on the label. The difference in the grades of olive oil can be seen in the color of the oil.

Extra-virgin olive oil is darker than the other types, and not as bright. Why is it better than the other types? It contains fewer chemicals and more antioxidants. It also has fewer free radicals. But researchers have found yet another reason why extra-virgin olive oil is superior to the other types (NDTV Food Desk, Updated: 2017, April 11).[83] Extra-virgin olive oil contains more hydroxytyrosol, which has the ability to reduce insulin resistance and non-alcoholic fatty liver disease.

But according to testing results published in late 2016, approximately 70 % of the olive oil available for sale in the United States is adulterated (Natural Cures House, 2017, February 13).[84]

Diluting olive oil with cheaper oils means that it could contain an oil that causes you to react, and the oil with which it is diluted certainly won't be listed on the label. That makes olive oil a relatively high risk item when trying to select a diet for recovery from an MC flare. It's a good choice for health benefits when it's pure, but not when it's adulterated with a cheaper oil. Oils such as sunflower or canola might be used, and that would simply limit the health benefits. But the oil used might be soy, which could cause a reaction for anyone sensitive to soy.

The probiotic fad.

Consumption of yogurt and other probiotic foods is popular today. Probiotic sales are brisk. Commercial yogurt sales are a multi-billion dollar business. Virtually everyone wants to have the same type of intestinal bacteria as one of the members of the hunter-gatherer tribes that existed a century or so ago in Tanzania, Venezuela, and Peru. They have been led to believe by their doctors and all the manufacturer sales pitches that not only would this improve their health, but they can achieve it by ingesting probiotics every day.

The reality is that it's not going to happen, because the only bacteria that are going to be able to attach to the intestinal walls and reproduce to establish a colony are the ones that previously occupied someone's gut and successfully attached there. The rest are all flushed away, despite what they may have cost. And they will continue to be flushed away as long as they are raised in a laboratory rather than someone's intestines.

But this is a pointless pursuit anyway, because everyone's gut bacterial profile is determined in the short term by the antibiotics they may have taken, and in the long term their microbiome is determined by their diet. So unless one eats exactly what those hunter-gatherers ate, the bacteria populations found in the intestines of hunter-gatherers are not going to survive in anyone else's intestine. If they are placed there, the population profiles will slowly shift to match the diet of the host. This is easily demonstrated. When people who have led a hunter-gatherer lifestyle are converted to a Western style diet, they soon develop a microbiome similar to everyone else who eats a Western style diet.

Comparing the gut biome of primitive hunter-gather tribes with ours might provide some interesting reading, but any information that comes from it is pretty much irrelevant. In 2016, the Los Angeles Times ran an article titled "The extinction inside our guts. Consider this quote from that article (Sonnenburg & Sonnenburg, 2016, February 25).[85]

> *Hunter-gatherers from Tanzania, Venezuela and Peru have a microbiota that is remarkably similar to one another and yet very different from ours in the West. Their guts harbor up to 50% more bacterial species and twice as many bacterial genes than ours do.*

Naturally the gut bacteria profile of most primitive tribes is similar — they are hunter-gathers and they hunt and gather basically the same foods. Obviously their gut bacteria demographics would have to be similar. And naturally their gut will provide housing for many more bacterial species — they have no refrigeration, no antiseptics or food preservatives. They don't even have plates on which to place their food. They're bound to eat a lot of things that you and I would never touch. So they would be likely to have much higher bacterial diversity in their guts, because of their lifestyle. But a comparison with our gut flora and fauna is irrelevant, because the bacteria populations in our guts are determined by our diet. If those subjects from hunter-gatherer tribes are fed the same diet we are eating, within a few months their gut biome will closely resemble ours.

The bottom line is that most, (maybe all) of the money spent on probiotics is wasted. Commercial probiotics, yogurt,, and similar products are going to end up being flushed down the toilet. They are not likely to change our microbiota for more than a few days.

The Los Angeles Times article reflects a common viewpoint to perpetuate the mistaken viewpoint that extinction is somehow an unnatural event. But the fact of the matter is that of all the species that have at one time or another existed on earth, 99.9 % are now extinct. And most of the extinctions occurred during five cataclysmic events. So extinction is a natural part of evolution. Is there any reason to believe that bacteria shouldn't be subject to the same laws of nature as the rest of us? Therefore it's natural for them to become extinct also.

The authors of such articles as that don't understand the human digestive system nor do they understand gut bacteria. Gut bacteria are simply opportunistic parasites who hang around as long as something in our gut appeals to them. If we change our diet and the item that attracted them disappears from their menu, they pack up and leave, to be replaced by new species of parasites who find the new diet appealing. It's that simple — survival of the fittest still rules in the human gut.

Researchers agree that probiotics are a waste of money for healthy adults.

A team of researchers at the University of Copenhagen looked at seven trials of probiotic products and they could find no evidence that the products altered the gut bacteria profile in healthy adults.[86] That said, some reviews have found that there is some evidence that in the case of individuals with bacterial imbalances due to certain diseases, a probiotic treatment regimen has been shown to be beneficial in some cases. Some of the evidence of treatment success is conflicting.

But since probiotics either do not help, or they make symptoms worse for most MC patients, and the American Gastroenterological Association Institute now expressly recommends against their use for the treatment of MC, probiotics are not only contraindicated for treating MC, but they have been found to be ineffective for altering the microbiome of healthy adults. This means that they are pretty much a product for which no practical use has been found, and like most other people, most MC patients are better off without them.

What about claims that when livestock or poultry eat gluten or soy in their feed it can show up in their meat?

Some authorities claim that soy (or gluten) can be transferred to the body of birds or animals. This is not in the medical literature because it has not been scientifically researched so the data have not been published, but logic says that the transfer of inflammatory peptides to the meat can only happen if those birds or animals experience incomplete digestion, because unless they have incomplete digestion, the final result of digestion is amino acids. Amino acids are not the cause of any known adverse reactions or intolerances. Allergic or intolerance reactions are caused by strings of amino acids, known as peptides that are somehow able to enter the bloodstream.

Peptides are the result of incomplete digestion. Incomplete digestion can be caused to one of two things — compromised digestion, or the inherent inability to digest certain items in the diet. In order for any peptides to enter the bloodstream, higher-than-normal levels of intestinal permeability must be present. And once peptides get into the bloodstream they will be deposited in joints, muscles, and various organs, much as happens with MC. This would make the peptides available in the processed meat.

And all this appears to be quite possible. There hasn't been any research conducted to verify that it happens, or to rule it out, so this is strictly speculative, but it certainly appears to be plausible. Incomplete digestion is certainly quite common, and disease or inflammation can cause leaky gut. In addition, fecal matter sometimes contacts the meat during the slaughtering process. That's counteracted by washing, and disinfectant rinses, but washing with water and disinfectant rinses does not always remove gluten residues, so the possibility of cross-contamination

91

during slaughtering, especially during the evisceration process, still exists in some situations.

The overall risk of having a reaction because of slaughter animal rations is probably low. It's difficult to ascertain the risk involved due to the lack of data on the prevalence of leaky gut among poultry or animals destined for slaughter, and data on possible gluten residues left on carcasses as a result of the evisceration process are unavailable.

Sometimes the failure of a recovery diet is due to trying to do too many things at once.

Some people find it impossible to stick with a diet long enough to get results. Because gluten and casein actually have the ability to be addictive (as we learned in the first edition of *Microscopic Colitis*), there may be withdrawal symptoms when they are excluded from the diet. Therefore some individuals may find it helpful to avoid multiple diet changes at the same time and instead, to make diet changes in multiple steps.

If gluten is removed from the diet first, this can often bring remission after a few weeks, and the remission will last for a few weeks until the immune system begins to react to the antibodies generated by other reactive foods in the diet. At that point all dairy products, or eggs, or products containing soy (or whatever food is thought to be a problem) can also be excluded from the diet. Subsequently other inflammatory foods can be removed until the diet is free of foods that are found to be or thought to be inflammatory. Some people find this easier to do than to cut all the inflammatory foods out at once, even though it might take longer to reach remission by doing this.

Anytime a diet is changed, the body has to make modifications to the digestive process. If slight diet changes are made, then only slight adjustments need to be made (automatically by the digestive system).

However, if drastic diet changes are made, then huge changes take place within the digestive system, especially regarding chemical changes (enzyme production changes). It takes a while for the digestive system to "learn" to produce more of certain enzymes, and to ramp up that production, especially for enzymes that have not been required in significant quantities previously. And this process becomes much more difficult if digestion is compromised by an IBD. The digestive system is like a complex manufacturing production line — it takes time to alter production methods, or to step up production quantities, especially if the machinery has mechanical problems. And whenever the diet is changed, the bacterial diversity and balance in the gut may change, which may also have some affect on digestion. All this suggests that making changes to the diet more gradually may have advantages in some cases.

But when inflammation is involved, the entire digestive environment is changed.

Inflammation interferes with enzyme production and therefore it interferes with digestion. It also interferes with absorption of nutrients. This results in huge shifts in the amount of partially-digested or undigested food moving through the digestive system. Undigested carbs, in particular, result in huge shifts in bacteria populations as opportunistic bacteria take advantage of all the partially-digested and undigested food available to them for fermentation in an ideal warm, moist, environment. So populations of bacteria attracted to rotting food can quickly build up. All of this typically happens before we change our diet to treat the disease.

So when we change our diet, our already-compromised digestive process is faced with additional changes (due to the removal of familiar foods, and the addition of unfamiliar foods). Initially, digestive efficiency may decline, because of the lag in the production of needed enzymes.

But as increased quantities of needed enzymes become available, and as the antibody levels and associated inflammation levels begin to come down, poorly-digested food becomes less available, so that populations of bacteria that are only there to help rot undigested food begin to decline. And eventually enzyme production and gut bacteria populations and balances will stabilize at an optimum level for the current diet as the digestive system continues to heal.

Any farmer or rancher will tell you that the diet of any animal should never be drastically changed, because that will often cause the animal to "go off feed" (stop or restrict eating, and lose weight), because of digestive system distress. Prudent livestock producers never make drastic changes to feed rations in a single step. They always make gradual changes over a period of a few days to a few weeks, depending on the extent of the diet changes that need to be made in the animal's ration.

For some people, cutting out gluten and dairy and possibly other foods may not be difficult, because those foods were not included in our evolutionary "ration" to begin with. But for most people who previously relied heavily on carbs and processed foods (which is virtually everyone, these days), the diet changes needed to heal the gut can amount to rather drastic changes. So perhaps it would be beneficial to use gradual diet changes, in order to cut our digestive system some slack when major diet changes need to be made.

If you're suspicious of a food, try this simple test.

A quick and simple way to detect foods that are likely to cause a reaction is to measure your heart rate before and after placing a sample of the food to be tested in your mouth and holding it there. The food will be immediately tested by your immune system through the mucosal tissues in your mouth and if you are sensitive to it, your heart rate will increase significantly. If your heart rate increases by more than about 10 % (usually about 6 or 7 beats per minute), you're probably allergic to that food. This isn't a sure-fire test, but it's sometimes helpful for making spur-of-the-moment decisions when eating out or whenever you have a reason to suspect cross-contamination.

And remember, the most difficult sensitivities to track down are the ones we eat every day, or are otherwise exposed to every day. This happens because when something becomes part of our regular routine it becomes a comfortable "old friend" and we learn to trust it.

Summary

In this chapter we found that there are many possible reasons why cross-contamination of the diet can prevent remission. These reasons include (but are not limited to) carelessness, mislabeling of processed foods, foods that are claimed by experts to be safe, but are actually not, loopholes in the labeling laws, natural flavors, fructose, vitamin E, product adulteration, cross-reactivity, and other causes.

Chapter 3

Nutritional Deficiencies

Most MC patients have vitamin and mineral deficiencies.

When asked about their diet, most people in the general population insist that they eat a healthy (nutritious) diet. And many do read labels and make a conscious effort to eat a relatively well-balanced diet that contains the nutrients that they need for good health. The health "experts", the FDA, and the USDA, tell us that if we follow their advice we will be healthy. But in the real world, health issues are becoming more prevalent and many diseases and associated nutrient deficiencies continue to increase. So where is the disconnect? Why isn't all this great advice working?

First off, some of the advice is either technically incorrect or intentionally misleading. It's based on obsolete or just plain incorrect information. Claims such as, "Animal fats should be avoided", or "When non-celiacs avoid gluten they unnecessarily put their health at risk", are just plain wrong. Animal fats are some of the healthiest fats available to us, because we evolved eating them. And there is certainly nothing wrong with anyone avoiding gluten. To the contrary, avoiding gluten is one of the best things anyone can do for her or his health.

And much of the advice is wrong by omission. Important vitamins and minerals that should be recommended, are not. So if we rely on "expert" advice for all our health information, we are likely to get a one-sided viewpoint. And we are doubly likely to accrue deficiencies of certain vitamins and minerals that become depleted because we have an inflammatory bowel disease.

How accurate is the nutritional information listed on most product labels?

Those labels may have been accurate several decades ago when the nutritional value of foods was first determined by USDA scientists (in the USA), but these days soils have become depleted after many decades of intensive farming and consequently many plants may not have the nutrients available to them that were available decades ago, especially magnesium. But we naively assume that most foods still contain the nutrient levels that they were found to contain decades ago. Do they?

Furthermore, if we look up the nutritional value of certain foods we find all sorts of values depending on the source of the information used, because all batches test differently. Who's information is right? It's all very confusing, and the bottom line is that we really don't know how accurate labeled nutritional information might be because it can vary so widely. So we just take their word on it, for better or for worse.

Nutrition labels constitute a manufacturer's guaranteed analysis. IOW the label guarantees that the product contains at least the amounts of those nutrients specified on the label. If they contain more, the excess is irrelevant (to the FDA).

But if the product actually contains less than the amount listed on the label, and someone alerts the FDA, the FDA will get all bent out of shape and send a letter to the manufacturer containing all sorts of ugly threats.

Most manufacturers try to understate the nutrient content of their products so that they don't have to worry about running afoul of the labeling laws in case any of the nutrients in an occasional batch happen to be at levels slightly below normal. So really, for all practical purposes, the FDA determines the nutrient levels listed on many labels.

To further complicate matters, many processed products are enriched with certain nutrients. Because most of those products tend to contain the cheapest forms of those nutritional supplements available, they may or may not actually provide any significant benefits for the consumer.

They meet FDA requirements, but that doesn't mean that anyone can actually utilize all of the nutritional supplements that are added. So it's no wonder that many people are not getting anywhere near the nutritional value from their food that they like to think they're getting.

For most people, magnesium needs are not being met today.

Doctors have forgotten how important magnesium is for health because these days they receive much of their ongoing education related to new treatments courtesy of their drug reps. And their drug reps never remind them of anything that doesn't require the use of expensive drugs. So traditional remedies that have worked since the beginning of human history tend to fall by the wayside, to be replaced by the use of new and expensive drugs. Over two decades ago Ma et al. (1995) showed that magnesium deficiency is associated with many serious long-term health issues, such as cardiovascular disease, hypertension, diabetes, insulin, and carotid arterial wall thickness.[87]

Writing about Dr. Norman Shealy, a well-known neurosurgeon and pioneer in the area of pain medicine, Dr. Mark Sircus pointed out that Dr. Shealy once noted that, "Every known illness is associated with a magnesium deficiency" (Sircus, 2009, December 8).[88] Dr. Shealy also noted that, "magnesium is the most critical mineral required for electrical stability of every cell in the body. A magnesium deficiency may be responsible for more diseases than any other nutrient."

Symptoms associated with a magnesium deficiency may include (but are not limited to) (Sircus, 2009, December 8):

- leg cramps
- foot pain
- muscle twitches or spasms
- constipation
- loss of appetite
- nausea
- vomiting
- fatigue
- weakness
- numbness
- tingling
- seizures
- twitches
- muscle tension
- muscle soreness
- back aches
- neck pain
- tension headaches
- urinary spasms
- menstrual cramps
- difficulty swallowing or a lump in the throat
- insomnia
- anxiety
- hyperactivity and restlessness with constant movement
- panic attacks

- agoraphobia
- premenstrual irritability
- personality changes
- abnormal heart rhythms
- coronary spasms
- palpitations
- heart arrhythmias
- angina due to spasms of the coronary arteries
- high blood pressure
- mitral valve prolapse
- irritability
- noise sensitivity
- hyper-excitability
- apprehensiveness
- an inability to control the bladder
- nystagmus (rapid eye movements)
- hearing loss
- osteoporosis.
- jaw joint (or TMJ) dysfunction
- chest tightness
- a peculiar sensation that one needs to take a deep breath but can't

The symptoms of severe magnesium deficiency may include:

- Extreme thirst
- Extreme hunger
- Frequent urination
- Sores or bruises that heal slowly
- Dry, itchy skin
- Unexplained weight loss
- Blurry vision that changes from day to day
- Unusual tiredness or drowsiness

- Tingling or numbness in the hands or feet
- Frequent or recurring skin, gum, bladder or vaginal yeast infections

Note that the symptoms of severe magnesium deficiency are also common symptoms of diabetes or what's known as prediabetes.

Normally, less than 1 % of our magnesium is located in our blood serum.

Yet when testing magnesium levels, most doctors naively order the serum magnesium test, presumably because it's quick and easy. But it's common knowledge that the serum test is woefully inaccurate. The National Institutes of Health list the important statistics for magnesium as follows.[89] Note the last sentence in the quote, which I have emphasized with bold print:

> *An adult body contains approximately 25 g magnesium, with 50% to 60% present in the bones and most of the rest in soft tissues. Less than 1% of total magnesium is in blood serum, and these levels are kept under tight control. Normal serum magnesium concentrations range between 0.75 and 0.95 millimoles (mmol)/L. Hypomagnesemia is defined as a serum magnesium level less than 0.75 mmol/L. Magnesium homeostasis is largely controlled by the kidney, which typically excretes about 120 mg magnesium into the urine each day. Urinary excretion is reduced when magnesium status is low.*
>
> *Assessing magnesium status is difficult because most magnesium is inside cells or in bone.* ***The most commonly used and readily available method for assessing magnesium status is measurement of serum magnesium concentration, even though serum levels have little correlation with total body magnesium levels or concentrations in specific tissues.***

Use the red blood cell (RBC) test rather than the serum magnesium test.

When testing magnesium levels becomes necessary, the most practical test to use is the RBC magnesium test. This blood test measures the amount of magnesium in red blood cells, which is representative of the amount of magnesium, found in many other cells in the body. While not a perfect test, it tends to be much more accurate than the serum test that's normally used. As an extreme example (if you have just taken a magnesium supplement, for instance), it's possible for a serum magnesium test to show a high, or even too high magnesium level, even though your RBC magnesium level (which is equivalent to the magnesium level inside your heart cells) might be so low that you are at risk of a sudden fatal heart attack.

And note that according to magnesium expert Dr Carolyn Dean (who has written several books about magnesium) and has her own highly-absorbable line of magnesium supplements, the so-called "normal range" of results even for the RBC test is inaccurate. She correctly points out that the "normal" results are based on a group of subjects who were 80 % magnesium deficient at the time, thus causing the results to be biased on the low side. She insists that the correct level for a normal test result should be 6.0–6.5 ng/ml (15–16.2 nmol/l), rather that the broad (and generally lower) range used by most laboratories.

Why are so many people magnesium deficient today?

Our ancestors drank water that supplied most of their magnesium needs because it came from streams, rivers, and lakes. As a result, we became accustomed to getting most of our magnesium from our drinking water. Surface water naturally contains high amounts of magnesium and other minerals because it washes over soils with relatively high mineral content. Today most people drink water that's filtered, aerated, and treated in other ways to remove minerals and various chemical contaminants. And, the soils have become depleted of many minerals because of intensive farming, so water moving over it is much less likely to pick up significant amounts of magnesium and other minerals than it did in the past. As a result, we have lost much of the magnesium in our drinking water, and virtually nothing has been done to replace those lost minerals.

It's claimed that only about 30 %-of the RDA of magnesium is available in two liters (the average amount needed for good health) of the water supplied by the cities where water contains the highest amounts of magnesium (Kiefer, 2007, February).[90] In most cities, only about 10 to 20 % of the RDA for magnesium is available in the water. And then on top of this many households don't trust the water supply, so they use additional filtering and water purification equipment which removes most of the remaining minerals. The amount of magnesium that's likely to get past these filtration systems is virtually zero (historyofwaterfilters.com, n.d.).[91]

Many people rely on bottled water for their drinking water. Bottled water varies greatly in purity, but sadly, except for some of the European brands, much of the water available in North America, both bottled and from the tap, contains very little magnesium (Azoulay, Garzon, & Eisenberg, 2001).[92]

This problem is greatly amplified by the general failure of the medical community to recognize and address the widespread magnesium deficiency that prevails among the general public. Part of the problem is that the so-called "normal" range for an acceptable magnesium blood level appears to be too low (Liebscher & Liebscher, 2004).[93] But the main problem is that the test universally used to test a patient's magnesium level (the serum magnesium test) is only very weakly associated with the actual magnesium level of the body. As we've already seen, the National Institutes of Health points out that less than one percent of the body's total supply of magnesium is available in blood serum, which makes this test a very poor indicator of the actual magnesium level in the body. Physicians are surely aware of this, and yet they blithely continue to use the test, mostly because it's cheap, easy, and traditional to use.

While the mainstream medical community continues to mostly ignore the problem, some believe that simply correcting magnesium deficiencies could eliminate many serious health problems, including heart disease and hypertension (Touyz, 2004).[94] It could also eliminate many less-serious but debilitating conditions. Many people believe, for example, that because so many fibromyalgia patients are magnesium deficient, fibromyalgia may be a symptom of magnesium deficiency (Deans, 2012, September 11).[95] Research has even been published showing that magnesium treats fibromyalgia (Engen et al., 2015).[96]

Women blame PMS symptoms on hormonal changes.

But during the second half of the menstrual cycle, when estrogen and progesterone levels go up, the magnesium level declines dramatically (Matthews, 2013, September 03). [97] This can cause spasms in the arteries that supply the brain with blood, resulting in PMS symptoms and migraines. But all of these symptoms can be reduced by significantly boosting magnesium reserves by increasing magnesium intake before the symptoms develop. It's common to crave chocolate before menses. This occurs because dark chocolate (with at least 80 % cocoa content) contains more magnesium than any other type of food. So are PMS symptoms due to hormonal changes, or are they actually due to a magnesium deficiency?

Why is magnesium deficiency such a big problem with microscopic colitis?

Approximately 11 % of magnesium is absorbed in the duodenum and 22 % is absorbed in the jejunum (Albion Laboratories, Inc., n.d.).[98] But about 56 % of magnesium is absorbed in the ileum and another 11 % is absorbed in the colon, both of which are inflamed in most MC patients (Albion Laboratories, Inc., n.d., Koskela, 2011).

That means that fully two-thirds of the magnesium absorption normally takes place in the ileum and the colon. The inflammation present there severely limits the absorption of magnesium, whether from food or supplements. Magnesium deficiency is the inevitable result. Even though magnesium is involved in managing the activity of over 350 enzymes and is used in over 80 % of the body's metabolic functions, it continues to be poorly understood and unappreciated by the medical community.

To add to the problem, magnesium intake goes way down with the onset of microscopic colitis. Most of the magnesium that we normally get in our diet is found in dark green, leafy vegetables. And of course when the gut is inflamed we cannot tolerate normal amounts of those vegetables.

Magnesium is important for proper immune system functioning.

Cojocaru, Cojocaru, Tănăsescu, Iacob, & Iliescu, (2009). have found that during and after episodes of major bacterial infections, magnesium levels show a significant decrease within a few days of the onset that persists for several weeks.[99] This suggests that magnesium is used at above normal rates by the immune system to fight bacterial infections. Because MC is often associated with major changes in gut bacteria balances, and bacterial infections have long been suspected of being a potential cause of the development of MC, the availability of adequate amounts of magnesium may be very important for facilitating recovery from the disease.

And importantly, magnesium reduces CRP levels.

In 2005, King, Mainous, Geesey, & Woolson proved that magnesium reduces cardiovascular risk by lowering C-reactive protein (CRP) results.[100] In the study, they showed that people who ingest less than the RDA for magnesium are significantly more likely to have an elevated CRP level. This implies that a magnesium deficiency is likely to increase one's CRP level. A year later King, Mainous, Geesey, Egan, & Rehman (2006) published another detailed paper on the research project concluding that in people with low dietary magnesium intake, supplementing by taking more than 50 mg of magnesium daily was associated with a lower likelihood of having an elevated CRP level.[101]

Certain common foods and certain medications are known to deplete magnesium.

As already discussed, because of the depletion of the magnesium content of many intensively-farmed soils, many foods today may not contain the amount of magnesium they are thought to contain. And some foods that are commonly a part of most diets today are known to actually hinder the absorption of magnesium or otherwise deplete it. Those foods were either not available during paleolithic times or were not commonly eaten during human evolution. Foods such as coffee, tea, carbonated drinks, sugar and sweet foods for example are known to deplete magnesium. Many medications either deplete magnesium or interfere with it's absorption, and obviously those medications were not available in paleo times. Examples are certain antibiotics, corticosteroids, and PPIs, all of which are known to severely deplete magnesium. And of course these medications are often prescribed for the treatment of MC.

Magnesium deficiency associated with the use of PPIs is such a major problem that the FDA has posted this warning about PPIs.[102]

> *[3-2-2011] The U.S. Food and Drug Administration (FDA) is inform-ing the public that prescription proton pump inhibitor (PPI) drugs may cause low serum magnesium levels (hypomagnesemia) if taken for prolonged periods of time (in most cases, longer than one year).* **In ap-proximately one-quarter of the cases reviewed, magnesium sup-plementation alone did not improve low serum magnesium lev-els and the PPI had to be discontinued.**

Note the last sentence in that warning especially (I have used bold print to emphasize it). If you take a PPI for an extended period, you almost certainly have a magnesium deficiency.

A general rule for recovering from MC is to re-cover first, correct deficiencies later.

When initially recovering from microscopic colitis, an important rule to remember is that correcting vitamin and mineral deficiencies in general is best left until after remission is achieved. The problem with trying to correct diet deficiencies during recovery is that many of the sup-plements available tend to contain ingredients that can prevent remis-sion in many cases, simply because they may add to the inflammation.

It's always much safer to wait until remission is achieved, and then if there is a valid reason why they are needed, supplements can be tried, one at a time, so that if they cause any problems, they can be immediate-ly identified and eliminated. Attempting to fix everything at once, be-fore remission is in place, often results in a long, drawn-out recovery process that may bring improvements, but never actually brings remission.

However, Magnesium and vitamin D are exceptions to that general rule because they are so important to healing. A magnesium or vitamin D deficiency should be corrected as quickly as possible, because adequate magnesium and vitamin D are vital to recovery, and there are plenty of safe sources for these supplements readily available.

We tend to think that if we eat a diet that provides all of the nutrients recommended by official government guidelines, we are doing all that we can to ensure optimum health. But the problem with this viewpoint is that the recommended RDAs of many nutrients may not actually be adequate for anything more than minimal protection against disease. For example, statistical evidence indicates that the range of acceptable blood levels of vitamin D (according to the guidelines) may only be adequate for the prevention of the disease known as rickets. A significantly higher level of vitamin D is necessary if one is concerned about minimizing the chances of developing other diseases (GrassRootsHealth, 2010, March 23).[103]

Taking supplements versus getting your vitamins and minerals from whole foods.

The human digestive system was designed to derive nutrition from whole food, where nutrients are typically diffused throughout the food. In many cases, the combinations of nutrients may offer synergistic effects that are not available in concentrated supplements. Humans evolved eating real food for over 2 million years. When food laboratories came along, innovative researchers decided that if food was nutritious for human health, then the individual nutrients in food must be the most important parts of food, and isolating them and utilizing them as supplements should be even better than eating whole food. At least that's the reasoning behind the concept of many vitamin and mineral supplements.

But in the real world, eating real food almost always provides far better long-term health than trying to get nutrition out of a bottle. The digestive system can extract nutrients from real food much more efficiently than from concentrated supplements. This is the reason why when supplements are taken, the doses have to be so much larger than the amount of nutrients defined by the RDA and provided by real foods. And what happens to all those excess nutrients that are absorbed from the supplements but not utilized by the body? They have to be removed from circulation by the liver or kidneys and purged from the body, possibly overloading these organs because they were not designed to do that on a full-time basis. That's not saying that supplements are always bad — when they are the only option, then they are obviously better than nothing. But they should not be viewed as a primary source of nutrition in the long run unless the digestive system is permanently compromised to a degree that food is no longer a reliable source of complete nutrition. Whenever possible, getting nutritional needs from food is far superior to taking supplements.

That said, there are a couple of exceptions to that general rule. Vitamins B-12 and folic acid may be absorbed more efficiently from the right type of supplements than from whole food, especially by individuals who have methylation issues. We'll look at methylation issues in the next chapter.

Types of magnesium.

There are many supplemental magnesium options to chose from. Choosing the right type can mean the difference between resolving a deficiency and just adding to the diarrhea. Magnesium is not stable in a pure state. In fact it's highly combustible when it's in a powdered state.

It can be more combustible than most common types of gunpowder, So it's always offered as a safe, stable compound when sold as a health supplement. Commonly-available magnesium compounds include (but are not limited to) these forms:[104]

> magnesium oxide
> magnesium chloride
> magnesium carbonate
> chelated magnesium (magnesium glycinate)
> magnesium orotate
> magnesium citrate
> magnesium maleate
> magnesium gluconate.

The percentage of magnesium available in these compounds varies, and so does the absorbability. For example for products intended to be absorbed through the skin, Ancient Minerals says that their products contain these amounts of elemental magnesium:[105]

> *Magnesium Oil: 560mg per teaspoon**
> *Magnesium Gel: 490mg per teaspoon*
> *Magnesium Bath Flakes: 15g per cup*
> *Magnesium Lotion: 185mg per teaspoon*
>
> **8 sprays of Magnesium Oil equals roughly 100mg of magnesium.*

Magnesium oxide is the most dense magnesium compound and the cheapest, so it is the one most often used in mineral supplements and multivitamins. It's also the type most often used by hospitals. It contains a lot of magnesium (300 mg of elemental magnesium per 500 mg tablet), but it's extremely poorly absorbed. At best, only about 4% of its elemental magnesium can be absorbed, making it a much better laxative than a magnesium supplement.

Magnesium chloride (soluble in water, and commonly found in sea water) is often used as a liquid to be sprayed or slathered on the skin, or as a bath or foot soak, whenever absorption of magnesium though the skin is desired. Magnesium chloride contains about 25 % elemental magnesium, but when in solution, the amount of available magnesium depends on the dilution. Magnesium carbonate contains about 125 mg of elemental magnesium per 500 mg tablet, but it is poorly absorbed.

Chelated magnesium (magnesium glycinate) is magnesium bound to the amino acids glycine and lysine. So it's easily absorbed and highly bioavailable. It usually contains 100 mg of elemental magnesium magnesium in each tablet. Most people find this to be a very good magnesium supplement.

Magnesium orotate contains only 31 mg of elemental magnesium per 500 mg tablet, but it's usually well absorbed. Magnesium citrate contains 80 mg of elemental magnesium per 500 mg tablet. It's much better absorbed than magnesium oxide, but higher doses can act as a laxative. Magnesium maleate is not commonly used, but it contains 56 mg of elemental magnesium per 500 mg tablet. Magnesium gluconate contains 27 mg of elemental magnesium per 500 mg tablet, and it's easily absorbed and quick acting. All forms of magnesium supplements are better absorbed when taken with food.

Magnesium Deficiency may be associated with cholesterol levels.

There is good evidence that magnesium lowers cholesterol and triglycerides (Massey, 2015, February 7, Rayssiguier, Gueux, & Weiser, 1981).[106, 107] In fact, for diabetes patients, cardiovascular issues are the main cause of death or illness. A diet rich in magnesium has been shown to provide cardioprotective effects (Olatunji, & Soladoye, 2007).[108] Conversely, magnesium deficiency can lower HDL cholesterol, at least this has been found to be true for people who have diabetes (Guerrero-Romero, & Ro-dríguez-Morán, 2000).[109] Magnesium can be life-saving when given in cases of myocardial infarction caused by an acute magnesium deficiency (Efstratiadis, Sarigianni, & Gougourelas, 2006).[110]

Depression is a common complaint among MC patients.

Eby and Eby, (2006) suggest that magnesium readily relieves depression symptoms.[111] Case studies show that magnesium supplementation usually brings fast recovery of depression symptoms, and in addition it often resolves many other health issues.

Magnesium can be beneficial for resolving many issues.

There is an association between stress, depression, anxiety, and tinnitus. The association is so common that in a high percentage of tinnitus cases, treating depression or anxiety issues can resolve, or at least significantly improve tinnitus symptoms.[112] Because of the association of tinnitus with anxiety and depression, there is some evidence that magnesium may be used as a treatment for tinnitus in some cases.[113] Research is underway to verify or disprove this concept.

Magnesium deficiency and Hashimoto's disease or hypothyroidism.

The leading cause of hypothyroidism in the U.S.A. is Hashimoto's disease, which is an autoimmune disease. Magnesium is important for the activation of thyroid hormone T4 (Kent, 2015, November 11).[114] Without adequate magnesium, T4 is not activated into the usable form, T3. Therefore, if one has a magnesium deficiency, even taking a T4 supplement such as levothyroxine sodium (Synthroid) is not likely to pro-

vide relief of symptoms. Many physicians do not understand that relationship — consequently they refuse to issue a prescription for a natural
desiccated product for treatment, mistakenly insisting that synthetic T4
should be a sufficient treatment. Of course they also fail to prescribe
magnesium, so their prescribed treatment does not work to relieve the
symptoms of many hypothyroid patients.

Magnesium deficiency is surely associated with MC in additional ways
that have not even been considered by researchers. In chapter 5 we will
look at how magnesium deficiency can cause inflammation on a cellular
level.

Magnesium deficiencies and iron deficiencies often occur together.

This is because magnesium and iron are often found together in the
same foods, so if your diet is short of one, it may be short of the other.
And the absorption of magnesium and iron seems to be synergistic.
That is, ingesting them together seems to result in better absorption of
both, compared with ingesting them separately. But the bottom line is
that if you are deficient of one, you are probably deficient of the other.
Having too much phosphorous in the diet can interfere with the absorption of magnesium, calcium, and iron.[115] If you are anemic, you are
probably also magnesium deficient. But correcting a magnesium deficiency is almost always easier to do than correcting an iron deficiency.
Correcting an iron deficiency while recovering from MC is tough to do,
because most iron supplements tend to cause digestive system upset.

An iron deficiency may be due to too much calcium in the diet. Calcium
is the only substance known to inhibit the absorption of iron in both
heme and non-heme form. But of course there are other foods or sub-
stances that can interfere with the absorption of one or the other form of
iron, such as cocoa, tea, and coffee.

When magnesium deficiency causes anxiety, in some cases it can cause breathing problems.

Anxiety tends to be self-sustaining, and the symptoms can be frightening. But how can we tell whether a breathing problem is due to anxiety, caused by a magnesium deficiency, or happening because of a heart or lung problem?

First we need to rule out any heart or long problems. Only a physician can do that.. She or he may not be able to pinpoint anxiety as the cause of the problem, but a doctor can certainly rule out a heart or lung issue. Once we're sure that our heart and lungs are not responsible for the problem, then we can proceed to verify that anxiety is the cause.

Breathing issues can be deceiving.

When anxiety becomes a problem, we tend to breathe faster. We may get the impression that we need to take in more air, so we try to take a deep breath. But we're unable to take a deep breath. So we try again. Again we're unable to draw a deep breath. It's natural to think that because we're unable to draw in a deep breath, we may not be getting enough oxygen. So we keep trying, unsuccessfully, to take a deep breath. And the more we try and fail, the more anxious we become.

But in reality, the reason why we can't draw a deep breath in the first place is because we're already taking in too much oxygen, not too little. We're actually short of carbon dioxide, not oxygen. We're hyperventilating. As our carbon dioxide deficiency becomes worse, we may experience other symptoms, such as chest pain, lightheadedness, muscle weakness, or tachycardia (rapid heartbeat). This situation is likely to lead to a classic anxiety attack (panic attack).

When we try to consciously control our breathing (to take a deep breath), we're practicing conscious breathing —we become conscious of every breath. As long as we breathe normally, this is all taken care of automatically. And we only take in as much oxygen as necessary — no more, no less than we need. But when we take conscious control of our breathing, we tend to take in more oxygen than we need (we naturally try to err on the safe side).

Because anxiety automatically tends to cause us to breathe more rapidly, it starts a cascade of events that may coerce us into believing that we actually have a breathing problem. And as we continue to attempt to draw a deep breath, thinking that will resolve the problem, pretty soon we do indeed have a breathing problem. We're hyperventilating, but we don't realize it.

Of course the solution is to take smaller breaths, and to breathe more slowly. Breathing in slowly (breathing through our nose), holding it for a while, and then breathing out slowly, should allow us to regain control of our breathing, and the symptoms should slowly fade.

Why do virtually all mainstream physicians fail to recognize the importance of magnesium?

Before we leave magnesium to go on to vitamin D, I'll offer this explanation of why mainstream medicine completely misses the boat when it comes to the importance of magnesium for good health. On their information page about magnesium, the University of Maryland Medical Center says in their very first paragraph:[116]

"Although you may not get enough magnesium from your diet, it is rare to be deficient in magnesium."

Say what? It's common knowledge that the majority of the population is magnesium deficient. Could the University of Maryland statement (that seems to contradict itself) illustrate the naivety of mainstream medicine any more precisely? Where do they think we're supposed to get our magnesium? If we don't get it from our diet, we're certainly not likely to absorb magnesium from the air we breathe.

Magnesium is used as a cofactor for converting the inactive form of vitamin D into the active form.

Published data tells us that if magnesium supplies are inadequate, the body will be unable to utilize vitamin D, because it will be unable to convert it from 25-hydroxyvitamin D [25(OH)D] into the active form of 1,25-dihydroxyvitamin D [1,25-(OH)2D] so that it can use vitamin D to fight inflammation and do all the other wonderful things attributed to vitamin D (Reddy & Sivakumar, 1974, Rude et al., 1985).[117, 118] This is old research, but it's vitally important for healing and long-term health, and modern medicine tends to completely ignore it. This probably defines why some patients are unable to reach remission. Healing is severely compromised if the patient has a magnesium deficiency, and if the deficiency is bad enough, recovery may be impossible despite meticulous attention to other treatment details. This clearly illuminates why magnesium adequacy is so important when attempting to recover from MC or any other IBD.

Be sure you stay hydrated — it's easy to become dehydrated when microscopic colitis is active.

Most people don't think of water as a nutrient, but water is essential for life and good health in general. Most people can survive for several months without food, if necessary, but without water, about 10 days is the survival limit. Experts insist that most people in the general population need to drink more water, and that's especially true for MC patients. Most doctors ordinarily fail to recognize a dehydration problem. According to Dr. Mark Sircus, one of the most common reasons for lawsuits in emergency room medicine involving pediatric patients is dehydration (Sircus, 2010, September 20).[119] Dehydration can occur surprisingly fast, especially when MC is active.

And when dehydration occurs, so does magnesium deficiency. This happens because dehydration tends to cause diarrhea, and electrolytes that would normally be absorbed during the digestive process cease to be absorbed when diarrhea becomes active. So electrolytes are lost with the diarrhea. And of course magnesium is one of the most important electrolytes lost.

When the diarrhea typically associated with microscopic colitis remains uncontrolled for long periods (a year or longer). the malabsorption problems that typically accompany chronic diarrhea can lead to serious vitamin and mineral deficiencies in many cases. In particular, deficiencies of vitamin D and magnesium are extremely common, but deficiencies of many of the B vitamins and other vitamins and minerals can also occur. Failure to address these issues in a timely manner can delay or prevent remission. And in some cases these unresolved deficiencies can increase the risk of a more serious relapse of symptoms upon accidental exposure to food allergens or cross-contamination of the diet.

Vitamin D deficiency is far more common than we would expect.

Because many foods are now fortified with vitamin D during processing, being so vitamin D deficient that we are at risk of developing rickets is no longer a common occurrence, but vitamin D deficiency is still widespread today in all ages groups (Pfotenhauer, & Shubrook, 2017).[120] More people stay indoors more of the time than they did years ago, so they tend to get less sun exposure. In addition, some medications and certain diseases (such as IBDs) interfere with the absorption of supplemental vitamin D, including vitamin D in food. Because vitamin D is utilized by the immune system when fighting disease, vitamin D tends to become depleted. For many reasons, most people today don't usually take in as much vitamin D as their ancestors did.

The fear of skin cancer and the overuse of sunscreen is at least partly responsible for the general public's tendency to be vitamin D deficient today. The most concerning issue is that the problem is becoming worse over time. Despite the fact that most people assumed that the vitamin D deficiency problem has been solved decades ago, the problem is very much with us today, and becoming worse with the passage of time. According to the National Health and Nutrition Examination survey, administered by the U. S. Government., data taken during the years between 1988 and 1994, showed that about 45 % of the public had a blood level of at least 30 ng/ml (75 mmol/l) (National Health and Nutrition Examination Survey. (2013, September 30, Ginde, Liu, & Camargo Jr, 2009).[121],[122]

30 ng/ml (75 mmol/l) is considered by many medical authorities to be the minimum acceptable level for vitamin D adequacy. Ten years later, the data show that only about half as many people (23 %) have at least the same blood level (30 ng/ml) (75nmol/l) of vitamin D (National Health and Nutrition Examination Survey. (2013, September 30, Ginde, Liu, & Camargo Jr, 2009). Needless to say, this trend must be corrected if an acceptable level of vitamin D for good health is to be maintained.

Vitamin D deficiency exists even in the most unlikely places.

Recently the American Academy of Orthopedic Surgeons conducted a research project that revealed that over half of the college football players were vitamin D deficient.[123] And of course this puts them at higher risk of injury to their bones and muscles. Why on earth should college athletes be vitamin D deficient? This illustrates the extent of the vitamin D deficiency problem.

In addition to not getting as much vitamin D from exposure of the skin to the sun, today we have many other possibilities that may lower blood levels of vitamin D. Research has shown how exposure to certain chemicals can lower vitamin D levels. Bisphenol A (aka BPA) is what is known as an endocrine-disrupting chemical (EDC), and EDCs have been shown to be capable of reducing vitamin D blood levels (ScienceDaily, 2016, September 20, Johns, Ferguson, & Meeker, 2016).[124, 125] EDCs are found in certain plastics and other items to which we may be exposed virtually every day. They are found in many personal care products and food packaging in the form of BPA and phthalates (ScienceDaily, 2016, September 20, Johns, Ferguson, & Meeker, 2016).

Vitamin D is present in the body in several forms.

Vitamin D supplements are available in the form of D2 and D3. In the body, sunlight (actually the ultraviolet B spectrum of sunlight) is used to convert an ever-present form of cholesterol (7-dehydrocholesterol), which is found in human skin, into D3. D3 can be measured in the blood, and the correct chemical designation is 25(OH)D3. Usually the trailing 3 is omitted because the vitamin D in the body is virtually always all D3 except for a very small fraction of D2, resulting in the chemical formula 25(OH)D. So if neither D2 or D3 is specified, it's almost always safe to assume that the reference is to D3.

But the immune system uses the active form of vitamin D (known as calcitriol) to defend us against disease and infection. When the active form is needed, 25(OH)D is converted into 1,25(OH)2D (calcitriol) by the kidneys. In the chemical formula for the active form of D [1,25(OH)2D] the last "2" refers not to D2, but to the fact that this form has two hydrogen and oxygen pairs. If you want to learn more about vitamin D, the Harvard Medical School does a good job of explaining the details (Vitamin D and your health: Breaking old rules, raising new hopes., 2007, February).[126] When a patient's vitamin D level is measured, it should always be measured as 25(OH)D, because this is the form in which vitamin D is stored in the body. The active form [1,25(OH)2D] is only produced as needed, so the level varies significantly.

What's the difference between vitamin D2 and vitamin D3?

Vitamin D2 is known as ergocalciferol. It is produced by plants and it's used to fortify some foods, because it's cheap. It's often prescribed by physicians when vitamin D deficiency is diagnosed. But the problem with D2 is that it's usually poorly absorbed by humans, compared with D3 (cholecalciferol). D3 is the predominant form found in humans and most other animals. Published research shows that D3 is more effective at raising blood levels of 25(OH)D (Tripkovic et al., 2012).[127]

Furthermore this study showed that daily dosing is far superior to weekly dosing. Other research has found that D3 is at least 3 times more effective than D2, for most common purposes regarding human health (Group, 2014, June 9).[128] So obviously D3 should be much preferred over D2. You will notice that when your own 25(OH)D levels are reported on tests, your D2 level is typically reported as less than four (<4 ng/ml [<10 nmol/l] unless D2 is being supplemented). It seems pointless that vitamin D2 levels are still reported, but old habits are hard to break, so the medical community continues to report D2 levels on tests, as if that were useful information

Since vitamin D2 plays such an insignificant role in human health, to simplify the way that information is presented in this book, vitamin D3 will be designated as simply "vitamin D" unless otherwise specified.

And conversely, whenever "vitamin D" is written, this can be assumed to stand for vitamin D3.

Magnesium should also be supplemented any time vitamin D is taken.

If the body does not have sufficient magnesium reserves, taking vitamin D can create a magnesium deficiency. Here's why that can happen. The body will utilize the additional vitamin D to absorb extra calcium from the diet. Magnesium is required (along with insulin) to transport the calcium from the bloodstream to its final destination in cells (in bones,or other organs) (Takaya, Higashino, & Kobayashi, 2004).[129]

If magnesium in the diet is inadequate to meet the demand, the needed magnesium is taken from body reserves (extra magnesium is usually stored in muscles). When that happens during the night, the magnesium is often taken from leg muscles, The result is usually leg and foot cramps, or sometimes what is known as "restless leg syndrome".

If the problem is excessive calcium (usually caused by taking too much calcium supplement), and the insulin and magnesium cannot meet the needs for transporting the calcium to where it can be used, then the extra calcium in the blood must be purged in order to maintain a normal calcium level in the bloodstream. Too much calcium in the blood (known as hypercalcemia), can lead to fatal coronary consequences. So the body is going to try to remove the excess calcium in the bloodstream. Removing it consumes more magnesium.

If insulin resistance is already a problem, then any extra magnesium in the blood also cannot be properly stored in the cells, so much of any excess may be purged by the kidneys, and therefore wasted, further depleting magnesium (Sircus, 2009, December 8).[130] Because of this interdependency, it's always a good idea to take a magnesium supplement any time we take vitamin D (Dean, 2012, August 15).[131]

Incidentally, the evidence against taking a calcium supplement (for any reason) is quite strong, A very large study involving about 24,000 men and women between the ages of 35 and 64 showed that those who took a calcium supplement more than doubled their risk of having a heart attack (Li, Kaaks, Linseisen, & Rohrmann, 2012).[132] Li, Kaaks, Linseisen, and Rohrmann (2012) showed that taking a calcium supplement increased the actual risk of heart attack among the men and women in the study by a surprising 139 %. By contrast, the amount of calcium in food made no difference in the risk.

The well known leader in functional and integrative medicine Chris Kressor has said this about calcium supplements, "That said, there are several supplements that are commonly recommended by conventional doctors and healthcare practitioners that are unnecessary at best, and potentially harmful at worst. Perhaps the best example of this is calcium".[133] In his blog he explains the details of why that's true.

Vitamin D is fat soluble.
The main reason we are likely to be vitamin D deficient in the first place (aside from the general malabsorption problem) is because vitamin D is fat soluble (not water soluble). Virtually all IBD patients have problems absorbing fat, this is why most MC patients are vitamin D deficient unless they take an adequate supplement. A significant amount of the vitamin D that might otherwise be available in our diet goes down the toilet with the unabsorbed fat.

Research has shown that vitamin D can be very beneficial when treating inflammatory bowel disease.

In a double-blind, randomized, placebo-controlled study, Raftery et al. (2015) showed that Crohn's disease patients have a lower CRP level (meaning less inflammation), fewer clinical symptoms, and a better quality of life in general as their vitamin D blood level increases in response to vitamin D supplementation.[134] Three months into the treatment the group that was taking vitamin D had developed a significantly higher blood level of vitamin D than the group taking the placebo. They had no indicators of leaky gut. The control group however, was found to have increased intestinal permeability. Apparently vitamin D treats leaky gut. This is a very important finding if it can be verified by other researchers. Unfortunately there doesn't seem to be any research in this area specifically directed at MC, but surely vitamin D has the same beneficial effect on inflammation associated with the other IBDs, including MC.

Furthermore, researchers have shown that relatively high doses of vitamin D can help Crohn's patients to stay in remission longer. In another random, double-blind, controlled study, Narula, Cooray, Anglin, and Marshall (2017) showed that patients taking a 10,000 IU daily dose of vitamin D were very resistant to relapse compared with patients who were taking 1,000 IU of vitamin D per day.[135] None of the patients taking the higher dose suffered a relapse during the 12-month duration of the study, compared with 38 % in the lower vitamin D rate group who had a relapse of symptoms. Similar to the study done by Raftery et al. (2015), the improvement in remission integrity by the group taking the higher dose of vitamin D apparently was due to the improved control of intestinal permeability. Blood levels of the patients taking the 10,000 IU dose increased from an average of 29 ng/ml (73 nmol/l) to 64 ng/ml (161 nmol/l) by the end of the 12-month study. Blood levels of the patients taking 1,000 IU of vitamin D increased from an average of 28 ng/ml (71 nmol/l) to 33 ng/ml (83 nmol/l) by the end of the study. About half the subjects in each group were already taking a vitamin D supplement when they enrolled in the study.

So could high doses of vitamin D3 be used to treat microscopic colitis? Maybe. There's good epidemiological evidence that MC can be treated by a combination of magnesium and vitamin D. This is in addition to the necessary diet changes, of course. Based on these research data for Crohn's disease patients, it appears that serum 25-hydroxyvitamin D [25(OH)D] levels above 40 ng/ml (100 nmol/l) might possibly be beneficial for all IBD patients.

And in view of published research, it also appears that IBD patients can safely take relatively high doses of supplemental vitamin D for extended periods without any undue risk of overdose problems. In the second study cited above (Narula, Cooray, Anglin, & Marshall, 2017), patients were treated with daily doses of 10,000 IU of vitamin D3 for 12 months, and the researchers reported that the treatment was well tolerated.

Nausea is a common complaint for many MC patients during a flare.

Nausea is often caused by dysmotility of the digestive system, particularly a failure of the stomach to empty in a timely manner. This causes partially digested food (chyme) to back up in the stomach. In the warm, moist environment in the stomach, the chyme can soon begin to ferment, producing nausea. This is often a symptom of diabetes, so the problem may be worse if the patient happens to have diabetes. While prescription medications can help, this problem can also be helped by taking vitamin D.

Understanding Microscopic Colitis

Similar to diabetes patients, people who have Parkinson's disease sometimes are troubled by gastroparesis (delayed emptying of the stomach) and compromised (slow) gastrointestinal functioning in general. Not only have Parkinson's patients been shown to typically be vitamin D deficient, but researchers have determined that intestinal dysmotility is negatively correlated with vitamin D levels in Parkinson's patients (Kwon et al., 2016).[136] That is to say, the lower their vitamin D level, the more likely they are to have problems associated with gastrointestinal motility. Vitamin D supplementation seems to resolve their motility issues.

This implies that vitamin D is able to resolve certain neurological issues that affect the digestive system. This is important, and it may suggest that vitamin D can undo some of the damage caused by neurological issues that are known to be a result of gluten-sensitivity associated with MC. Of course at this point, this is just speculation, as no research has been done to either verify or to rule out it's possible relevance for microscopic colitis.

Recent research even suggests that vitamin D deficiency increases the risk of developing Alzheimer's disease (Mokry et al., 2016).[137] Apparently vitamin D has far-reaching effects on the brain and the central nervous system — far greater effects than are commonly recognized in the mainstream medical community.

But to get back to our original point, we have evidence that supplementing with vitamin D may help to resolve the nausea in vitamin D deficient patients that often accompanies MC and other inflammatory bowel diseases. We know, for example, that ulcerative colitis (UC) patients are more likely to suffer a relapse of symptoms if they are vitamin D deficient. In a physician-blinded research study of UC patients in remission, Gubatan et al., (2017) determined that vitamin D blood levels at or below 35 ng/ml (87 nmol/l) increased the risk of clinical relapse.[138] That suggests that maintaining one's blood level of vitamin D above 35 ng/ml (87 nmol/l) might be a prudent policy to follow with any type of IBD.

Medications are more effective when vitamin D is not deficient.

Increasingly, gastroenterologists are prescribing anti-tumor necrosis factor-α (anti-TNF-α) drugs to treat Crohn's and UC. This class of drugs works by suppressing the immune system of the patient Winter et al. (2017) showed that anti-TNF-α drugs are less likely to bring remission in vitamin D deficient patients.[139] In a study of Brigham and Women's IBD Center data for patients who were treated with anti-TNF-α medications, Winter et al. (2017) found that having vitamin D sufficiency carried increased odds of 2.64 of reaching remission within 3 months when compared with patients who were vitamin D deficient.

Vitamin D controls lipid balance.

In a 5-year study of over 13,000 people , Faridi et al., (2017) showed that those who were vitamin D deficient had a significantly higher risk of dyslipidemia than those who had a sufficient level if vitamin D.[140] Dyslipidemia is defined as having an elevated level of low-density lipoprotein (LDL), a low level of high-density lipoprotein (HDL), or a high total cholesterol (TC) level.

Research shows that the body uses what are known as sterol regulatory element-biding proteins (SREBPs) to create and transport cholesterol and fatty acids (Asano et al., 2017).[141] SREBPs are activated to increase the expression of the genes that are required to create the necessary enzymes whenever more lipids are needed. But if SREBP activity is excessive, the result can be various metabolic diseases including atherosclerosis, fatty liver disease, high cholesterol, insulin resistance, and obesity.

The activation of SREBPs is regulated by a feedback loop in which SREBPs are bound by a SREBP cleavage-activating protein (SCAP), which acts as an essential escort for activation purposes. Asano et al. (2017) showed that 25(OH)D degrades SCAP, thus making it an inhibitor of SREBP activation. The implications of this are that vitamin D might somehow be used to prevent or treat metabolic diseases.

Even many doctors have a chronic vitamin D deficiency.

This is probably why many physicians don't seem to be concerned about their patients' blood levels of vitamin D. They aren't even concerned about their own vitamin D level. Which suggests that they don't realize the importance of vitamin D for proper immune system functioning.

A study of Indian Doctors for example revealed that a majority of them are vitamin D deficient (Kalra, (2016, July 1).[142] That's probably why 69 % of Indians are deficient in vitamin D, and another 15 % are rated as insufficient.

India is situated where it is exposed to plenty of sunshine, but apparently, as is the case in the rest of the world, not very many people are taking advantage of that sunshine to maintain their vitamin D level. It's likely that if additional studies were done on American or European doctors' vitamin D levels, the results would be similar.

The problem seems to be worldwide, and is especially widespread among people who have digestive issues. In Saudi Arabia, a study of IBS patients showed that 82 % had a vitamin D deficiency (Khayyat & Suzan, 2015).[143] The problem has become serious enough in the U.S. that the Food and Drug Administration decided several years ago to add vitamin D to the labeling requirements for processed foods (Wilson & Christensen, 2014, February 27).[144]

Often, correcting nutritional deficiencies associated with an IBD can also resolve long-standing AI issues such as asthma.

In a randomized, double-blind, placebo-controlled trial, Tachimoto et al., (2016) showed that when added to a regular treatment program, low-dose, short-term supplementation with vitamin D brings improved asthma control in Japanese schoolchildren.[145]

Vitamin D has been shown to reduce chronic lower back pain (Ghai et al., 2017).[146]

Lower back pain is a common complaint when MC is active. The fact that vitamin D treats lower back pain is not surprising, considering it's record of helping to build bone and muscle mass. Even obstructive sleep apnea has been shown to be associated with vitamin D deficiency (Bozkurt et al., 2012).[147] These two seemingly unrelated events may not be unrelated, after all.

Another good reason to keep one's vitamin D blood level well up in the "sufficient" range is the risk of developing Alzheimer's disease.

Mokry et al. (2016) proved that certain gene mutations are associated with an increased risk of the development of Alzheimer's disease, and the increased risk is proportional to one's vitamin D blood level.[148] In other words, the lower the vitamin D level, the greater the risk of developing Alzheimer's disease.

How much vitamin D do we get from various sources?

Many studies have been published showing that we usually get around 120–180 IU of vitamin D per day from our food. Some studies show that we get more. That's not much. The Vitamin D Council says that everyone needs about an average of 5,000 IU per day.[149, 150] How much do we really get from our food, and how much do we get from the sun? Heaney, Armas & French, (2013) looked at eight such studies in an effort to evaluate studies made in typical situations in various developed countries of the world.[151] They found that the average total intake of vitamin D in these studies was about 2,200 IU per day. This resulted in average blood levels in the range of 20–25 ng/ml (50–62 nmol/l). They found that the average contribution from sunlight was only around 320–480 IU per day. Using conventional allowances for the amount of vitamin D in food, they found that food only contributed about 120–160 IU per day. That means that food and sunlight together only supply an average of about 400–600 IU per day. That leaves at least roughly 1,600 IU per day unaccounted for. Obviously that additional vitamin D must be coming from undocumented food sources (Heaney, Armas & French, 2013). Heaney, Armas & French, (2013) concluded that this discrepancy in the amount of vitamin D attributed to food may be due to the fact that meat contains 25(OH)D, and this source of vitamin D has been ignored in previous studies. If true, this would mean that the vitamin D contribution we get from our diet is much larger than previously recognized. It implies that we are only getting about 10–25 % of our vitamin D needs from the sun during the summer when the availability of solar energy peaks, and of course we're getting less during the rest of the year.

But the point is that this only gets us to an average blood level of 20–25 ng/ml (50–62 nmol/l). The Vitamin D Council recommends a blood level of Vitamin D in the range of 40–80 ng/ml (100–200 nmol/l) for optimal health.[152] Our paleo ancestors evolved to get a much larger share of vitamin D from the sun. And this is still seen in native equatorial populations where traditionally-living people get much more of their vitamin D from the sun than from their food. Clearly, either we need to get much more sun exposure, or we have to take a vitamin D supplement, or both.

How much vitamin D can we get from the sun?

Researchers in Spain estimated how much vitamin D we can expect to get from exposure to sunlight (Serrano, Cañada, Moreno & Gurrea, 2017, Fuentes, 2017, March 7).[153, 154] They determined that at mid-latitudes during the spring and summer months we can produce about 1,000 IU of vitamin D in 10 minutes if approximately 25 % of the body's skin surface is exposed to the sunlight. So if you want to generate the daily need of 5,000 IU, that would take about 50 minutes.

But the catch is that the researchers found that exposure for longer than 29 minutes significantly increased the risk of sunburn. So to get around that caveat you're going to have to expose more skin. But about 50 % is the practical limit (one whole side of the body). This would double the vitamin D production rate, and if you go the limit (3 x 10 minutes), you could safely produce about 6,000 IU of vitamin D. But we know that in the real world, people are able to exceed that amount regularly.

According to the Vitamin D Council, we can get from 10,000 to 25,000 IU of vitamin D from less than 30 minutes of sun exposure before our skin starts to burn.[155] But that depends on whether we are on a beach in Miami Florida, or a backyard in Calgary, in Alberta, Canada. Getting very much vitamin D from the sun is not going to happen in Calgary. And even in Miami, we may have to work at it to get enough vitamin D from the sun. It's not likely to happen accidentally, unless our job involves working out in the sun much of the day virtually every day. For most of us, therein lies the problem.— we can't get enough sun exposure unless we make a special effort to do so, regularly.

Furthermore, Serrano, Cañada, Moreno & Gurrea, (2017) determined that in January, with 10 % of the skin surface exposed, it took an average of 130 minutes to produce 1,000 IU of vitamin D. Sunburn risk came after about 150 minutes. They found that during the fall, in October, about 30 minutes of exposure time was required to produce 1,000 IU of vitamin D, with 25 % of the skin exposed.

All these times are for individuals who have a medium skin type and any color eyes and hair. Times would obviously vary for lighter or darker skin types, and of course times would vary with air quality or clouds, since those factors would affect sunlight intensity. So the problem is that for most of us, these days we're not likely to get enough sun exposure to get our vitamin D needs from the sun unless we especially go out of our way to make sure that we get the sun exposure we need. And even so, in the winter months our vitamin D level is likely to decrease, as the sun intensity declines because of the physical relationship of the earth with the sun. We may find it necessary to boost our vitamin D blood level with oral or topical supplementation, especially during the winter months, and especially if we live at a northern latitude.

Consider the factors that limit our ability to get vitamin D from sunlight.

To convert the 7-dehydrocholesterol in our skin into vitamin D requires that we allow sufficient time for the chemical transformation to take place. Conversion is a time-dependent process that takes approximately 48 hours for completion. Almost everyone showers or takes a bath more frequently today than people did a hundred or even fifty years ago and that's one of the reasons why we're no longer getting much of our vitamin D from sun exposure If we wash away the oily substance that's left on our skin after exposure to the sun, we're washing away the intermediate stage of the conversion, which means that what we're washing away, would have become vitamin D, given enough time. A light rinsing with plain water may not remove all of the material, but a vigorous scrubbing with soap and water will almost surely remove all of it and stop the conversion process. What would have become vitamin D will go down the drain.

When using sun exposure to generate vitamin D, there are many limiting factors. According to The Vitamin D Council (n.d.) we should consider these limiting factors:

1. Time — during the middle of the day sunlight is much more intense than at other times.

2. Location — the closer we are to the equator the more intense the sunlight.

3. Pigmentation — light-colored skin takes less time to produce a given amount of vitamin D.

4. Area — the larger the skin surface area exposed to the sun, the greater the amount of vitamin D we can produce.

5. Age — as we age, we are usually less able to produce vitamin D.

6. Sunscreen — obviously sunscreen blocks sunlight so it is contraindicated for vitamin D production.

7. Altitude — sunlight is more intense at higher altitudes, which enhances vitamin D production.

8. Clouds — sunlight is scattered by clouds, which reduces the amount of sunlight that is available to make vitamin D.

9. Pollution — air pollution scatters light, similar to clouds, which reduces the potential for making vitamin D.

10. Glass — glass blocks ultraviolet B light, which is needed to produce vitamin D

Note that while there is evidence that vitamin D raises cholesterol, sunlight exposure does not.

As we've already noted, supplemental vitamin D raises cholesterol. Recent research shows that when vitamin D is increased by additional sunlight exposure, compared with increasing 25(OH)D levels by taking vitamin D supplements, cholesterol levels are reduced, instead (Patwardhan et al., 2017).[156]   With increased sun exposure, Patwardhan et al. (2017) showed that total cholesterol (TC), low-density-lipoprotein (LDL), and high-density-lipoprotein (HDL) were all significantly decreased with 25(OH)D level increases due to increased sun exposure. Conversely, they showed that boosting vitamin D levels by taking conventional vitamin D supplements increased both TC and HDL, but only caused an insignificant increase in LDL levels.

How long should someone wait after changing the dosage before retesting vitamin D?

According to the Vitamin D Council, the "washout" period for vitamin D is considered to be about 10 weeks (Tovey, 2016, October 21).[157]   In other words, if someone stops taking vitamin D, or lowers the dose, after 10 weeks that person's 25(OH)D blood level should return to about where it was before starting to take vitamin D or before decreasing the dose.

Likewise, when increasing the dose, the blood level should be stabilized at the new level fully reflecting the dose change in about 10 weeks.

How should oral vitamin D be taken?

Published research shows that high weekly doses are counterproductive (Owens et al., 2017).[158] In one particular study, one group of athletes took 35,000 IU of vitamin D per week, while another group took 70,000 IU weekly (in one weekly dose) (Owens et al., 2017). While the 25(OH)D and 1,25(OH)2D3 (activated vitamin D) levels increased for both groups, the second group (taking the higher rate) began to produce increasing amounts of an enzyme that deactivates vitamin D. Apparently their bodies were attempting to maintain a balance and the higher dose exceeded the threshold with which the body was comfortable. Consequently the group taking the higher dose experienced a reduction in activated vitamin D, implying that their bodies were less able to perform important biological functions. This negative effect even continued for several weeks after taking the vitamins was stopped. Because of the lingering effect of lowered activated vitamin D levels due to the persistence of the production of vitamin D deactivating enzyme, higher doses of vitamin D should not be stopped abruptly. Instead, they should be tapered over a period of several weeks to give the body time to adjust. Whether due to deficiency, or excess supplementation, chronic depressed levels of activated vitamin D in the cells of the body can lead to increased risk of disease or other health issues. The evidence suggests that taking vitamin D daily is much preferred to taking an equivalent amount weekly (taking 7 times the daily dose at one time each week).

For some patients, vitamin D in liquid or oral spray form may be preferred.

Patients who have MC typically have an intestinal malabsorption problem, so they are always looking for ways to get around this issue when supplementing vitamin D or other nutrients. This might be a situation where oral sprays might be more effective, as they would bypass the intestinal malabsorption issue.

In comparison trials, oral vitamin D sprays have been shown to be as effective as oral capsules (Todd et al., 2016) [159] In a side by side comparison trial, where one group took capsules containing 3,000 IU of vitamin D daily, and another group used an oral spray, results were very similar. After 4 weeks of treatment the difference in serum levels of vitamin D in both groups was found to be close enough to be considered equivalent, for most practical purposes.

Subjects in both groups started the trial with an average serum vitamin D level of 23 ng/ml (57 nmol/l). At the end of the trial, the group using capsules showed an average vitamin D level of 36 ng/ml (90 nmol/l), and the group using the oral spray averaged 34 ng/ml (85 nmol/l).

Topical application of vitamin D is also effective.

Sadat-Ali, Bubshait, Al-Turki, Al-Dakheel & Al-Olayani, (2014) demonstrated that vitamin D can be supplemented effectively by applications to the skin.[160] In a trial involving the delivery of vitamin D in an aloe vera-based cream, compared with using the cream without vitamin D, they were able to raise the average 25(OH)D levels of the study group from 12 ng/ml (30 nmol/l) to 38 ng/ml (95 nmol/l), while the blood levels of the control group remained at an average of 11 ng/ml (27 nmol/l).

How much vitamin D is too much?

Note that it is impossible to get too much vitamin D by natural means. We cannot get too much vitamin D from sun exposure (but it's certainly possible to get sunburn from too much sun exposure) and we can't get too much vitamin D from eating unprocessed foods. I specified unprocessed foods because today, vitamin D is added to some processed foods by FDA mandate.

As it turns out, in many situations the added vitamin D is not likely to matter because much of the supplementation is in the form of D2, which is not well absorbed by most people anyway. And even in the cases where vitamin D is added in the form of D3, the amounts added are so small as to be no threat to the possible risk of an overdose for virtually everyone.

But it is possible to take too much supplemental vitamin D. We've already discussed the negative effects of taking individual large doses of vitamin D (compared with taking regular smaller daily doses). Regardless of how any supplemental vitamin D is taken, blood levels that exceed 150 ng/ml (375 nmol/l) are considered to be an indication of too much vitamin D (The Vitamin D Council, n.d.).[161]

This usually (but not always) happens as a result of taking 40,000 IU or more of vitamin D daily for more than three months. The risk is a state of hypercalcemia, which can lead to fatal cardiac events, so it's prudent to keep 25(OH)D levels below 150 ng/ml (375 nmol/l) This can happen because vitamin D can cause the absorption of more calcium than can be effectively regulated in the blood, particularly in the event of magnesium deficiency.

Remember that one of the functions of magnesium as a electrolyte is to remove excess calcium from the blood. If the blood level of calcium gets too high, it can lead to adverse cardiac events (including cardiac arrest).

Mainstream medical institutions post all sorts of dire warnings about taking vitamin D.

The following quote comes from one of the web pages on the Mayo Clinic website, for example.[162] Apparently these warnings are offered as advice to physicians.

> *Vitamin D may cause allergic skin reactions (inflammation, irritation, rash, and thinning), build-up of calcium in the arteries, changes in cholesterol levels, daytime sleepiness, excessive vitamin D levels, hardening of the arteries, headaches, increased calcium excretion or levels, increased risk of falls and fractures, increased risk of heart attack and stroke, increased risk of high blood pressure during pregnancy, increased risk of urinary tract infection, kidney or urinary stones, muscle pain, respiratory tract infection, and stomach problems (constipation, cramps, diarrhea, upset stomach, and vomiting).*

> *Vitamin D may affect blood sugar levels. Caution is advised in people with diabetes or low blood sugar, and in those taking drugs, herbs, or supplements that affect blood sugar. Blood sugar levels may need to be monitored by a qualified healthcare professional, including a pharmacist, and medication adjustments may be necessary.*

> *Vitamin D may affect blood pressure. Caution is advised in people with blood pressure disorders or those taking drugs or herbs and supplements that affect blood pressure.*

> *Use cautiously in people with headaches, heart disease, immune disorders (including lymph cancer and tuberculosis), kidney disease, liver disease, lung disorders, musculoskeletal disorders, skin disorders, stomach disorders, and thyroid disorders.*

Use cautiously in pregnant women at risk of high blood pressure associated with pregnancy.

Use cautiously in breastfeeding women.

Avoid in people with known allergy or sensitivity to vitamin D, any similar compounds, or any part of the formula.

Avoid in people with abnormal calcium excretion or levels.
Pregnancy and Breastfeeding

Use cautiously in pregnant women at risk of high blood pressure associated with pregnancy. The recommended adequate intake for pregnant women is the same as for non-pregnant adults. Most prenatal vitamins provide 400 IU of vitamin D daily as cholecalciferol, while high-risk populations may benefit from higher amounts (2,000-4,000 IU daily).

Use cautiously in breastfeeding women. The daily recommended intake for vitamin D during breastfeeding is 400 IU (10 micrograms) daily. Vitamin D2 in doses of 2,000 IU daily or 60,000 IU monthly for three months has been found to be safe and effective. Exclusively breastfed babies may be supplemented with 400-2,000 IU daily.

On the surface, these claims appear to be a major indictment of vitamin D for various health reasons. But if the claims are looked at individually, from an analytic viewpoint, it becomes clear that every one of them is associated with taking vitamin D when magnesium is deficient. We've previously established that unless one is already taking a magnesium supplement, significant doses of supplemental vitamin D should always be accompanied by a magnesium supplement. But of course since the Mayo Clinic and all other mainstream medical institutions turn a blind eye to the entire magnesium deficiency situation, they choose to blame taking vitamin D for problems that are due to magnesium deficiency.

And of course in the long run this results in fewer people taking a vitamin D supplement, which makes them more vulnerable to many pathogens that could otherwise be easily managed by their immune system.

In particular, physicians warn against 25(OH)D levels that are significantly above the industry-accepted standard of 30 ng/ml (75 nmol/l).

They apparently assume that the lack of research data in that range somehow indicates negative consequences. Accordingly, they seem to feel that the 40–80 ng/ml (100–200 nmol/l) range recommended as optimum for most people by the Vitamin D Council is too high, despite the fact that numerous research studies show that level to be associated with health benefits for most people. So few people in developed countries have a blood level of vitamin D above 40 or 50 ng/ml (100 or 125 nmol/l) these days that whenever a study is done, no conclusions can be drawn about higher doses because of insufficient data. So physicians continue to assume that because there is no research data, higher levels of vitamin D must be bad.

Yet even research on patients with IBS symptoms shows that symptoms are significantly improved after treatment with relatively high doses of vitamin D (Abbasnezhad et al., 2016).[163] So why does this seemingly industry-wide bias exist against the use of vitamin D to improve health? If we look at the list of possible negative effects that are often attributed to vitamin D, they typically include items such as heart attack, stroke, kidney stones, headache, nausea, vomiting, diarrhea, anorexia, weight loss, and low bone density, (osteoporosis).

But wait — we've seen those symptoms before. They're the symptoms of magnesium deficiency, a syndrome that's not even on the radar of most mainstream physicians. Out of all the symptoms listed, only diarrhea is truly a symptom of vitamin D toxicity. The rest are symptoms of magnesium deficiency. But we're not talking about vitamin D levels that are in the toxic range here — that would be 25(OH)D levels in excess of 150 ng/ml (375 nmol/l). Were talking about vitamin D levels about half that amount, or less. Perhaps the lack of understanding of the relationship between vitamin D and magnesium explains the bias.

Vitamin A may have an indirect effect on MC.

Estimates of the percentage of the population that is hypothyroid range from 5 % to about 20 %, depending on how one interprets the range of TSH values that the medical community considers to be normal. The range of TSH values currently considered to be normal by most medical professionals is typically about 0.5–5.0, but many authorities dispute this and claim that the normal TSH range should be 0.3–3.0.[164] According to an informal poll among members of an MC discussion and support forum, MC patients may be about 3 to 10 times as likely to have hypothyroidism, when compared with the general public, again depending on how "normal" TSH values are interpreted (Persky, 2008, June 4).[165] Farhangi, Keshavarz, Eshraghian, Ostadrahimi, & Saboor-Yaraghi, (2012) have demonstrated that vitamin A is capable of increasing T3 and thereby decreasing TSH values.[166] This can reduce hypothyroid effects. Therefore we don't have any direct proof, but there is a possibility that MC patients may benefit from vitamin A supplementation, particularly if they are having hypothyroidism symptoms.

But as we noted in the first book (*Microscopic colitis*), retinoic acid, which is a metabolite of vitamin A, together with interleukin-15 (IL-15) in the intestines of patients with celiac disease, has been shown by DePaolo et al, (2011) to possibly cause the inflammation that results in celiac disease.[167] Unless those research findings are proven to be false, it may be prudent to restrict any vitamin A supplements that might be taken, especially during recovery, to forms based on beta-carotene. Any form that contains retinol or retinoic acid might possibly cause problems in the event that this inflammation risk might apply to MC patients.

Vitamin B-12 reserves are usually stored by the liver for periods of up to about five years.

Consequently the malabsorption problem associated with MC is not likely to cause a B-12 deficiency unless the disease is not controlled promptly and clinical symptoms continue for more than about five years Of course there are exceptions, such as patients who are following or who have followed a vegetarian or vegan diet in the near past. Most plants contain very little vitamin B-12, so that anyone following a plant-based diet may be vitamin B-12 deficient, unless they have made a practice of routinely taking a vitamin B-12 supplement.

Folic acid is needed in order for vitamin B-12 to be properly utilized in the body, so if a vitamin B-12 supplement is taken, then a folate supplement should usually be taken also, to make sure that an adequate amount of folic acid is available to facilitate the use of a vitamin B-12 supplement.

What if my vitamin B-12 tests out-of-range?

Some people who take a vitamin B-12 supplement because they think their level may be low, find that when tested, their vitamin B-12 level will test surprisingly high. This may be because like most vitamins, B-12 is present in a number of different forms in the body and supplementation is likely to distort the balance between the various forms. It's necessary to stop taking a B-12 supplement and wait about a week to ten days before having a blood draw performed for a Vitamin B-12 test. This will allow the various forms of the vitamin to reach homeostasis (equilibrium), and the blood test result will be more accurate.

About half the population may have methylation issues because of a genetic mutation. Their B test results will usually be high-normal or above range, because their body is unable to properly convert the inactive forms of vitamins into the active forms so that their body can use them for various chemical transformations. Those individuals often benefit from taking the active forms of the "B" vitamins.

In the case of vitamin B-12, the form usually used in the cheaper vitamins is inactive and it's known as cyanocobalamin. Methylcobalamin is an active form which is much more readily absorbed, and this is the form that MC patients should use to get around their intestinal malabsorption problem. Methylcobalamin (combined with folic acid) is available in sublingual form, designed to be dissolved under the tongue, where it is absorbed directly into the mucosal tissues of the mouth.

For individuals who have methylation issues, taking the active form of vitamin B-6 may be beneficial.

Vitamin B-6 is also known as pyridoxal 5'-phosphate (P5P). At least a hundred chemical processes in the body depend on it. IBDs tend to deplete diamine oxidase (DAO) levels. As we discussed in the first edition of *Microscopic Colitis*, DAO appears to be the enzyme primarily used by the body to purge unused or excessive amounts of histamine in circulation, in order to prevent the possibility of a potentially harmful histamine buildup. One of the many uses of P5P is to promote the production of DAO enzyme. So P5P supplementation may be beneficial in cases where a DAO deficiency develops.

Vitamin B-2 (riboflavin):

A riboflavin deficiency is not recognized by the mainstream medical community as being associated with MC or any other IBD. However, vitamin B-2 is necessary in order for the human body to be able to utilize the energy in fats (and other nutrients). Riboflavin is used by the digestive system for metabolizing the energy held in proteins, fats, and carbs and converting it into a form of energy that the body can use.

A vitamin B-2 deficiency is quite common with anorexia and alcoholism. The reason why a vitamin B-2 deficiency might develop with anorexia is rather obvious, due to the nature of the condition, which interferes with the utilization of many nutrients in the diet. But the association with alcoholism is not as obvious. The common link with MC is intestinal permeability. Alcohol has been recognized for years as a primary cause of leaky gut.

Perhaps a vitamin B-2 deficiency is at least partially responsible for the overwhelming fatigue and lack of energy that are so often associated with MC. And maybe a vitamin B-2 deficiency is at least partially to blame for the persistence of fatigue symptoms as much as a couple of years past the achievement of remission, in many cases. Other than B-12, B-9 (folic acid), B-6, and B-2, normally, the other "B" vitamins are less likely to be potential problems for MC patients. That said, in a few cases they might be deficient

Migraines are often associated with MC flares.

Research has revealed that migraines are often associated with deficiencies in magnesium, vitamin D, co-enzyme Q10, and vitamin B-2. Certain medications, such as tricyclic antidepressants (such as amitriptyline) and anticholinergic medications (such as Benedryl) and others are known to interfere with the absorption of riboflavin or otherwise deplete the riboflavin level in the body.

Zinc deficiency is not common, but when it occurs, one of the symptoms can be diarrhea.

Zinc deficiency is associated with many intestinal diseases, because a zinc deficiency can compromise the ability of the tight junctions in the epithelia to function properly (Skrovanek et al., 2014).[168] A failure of this barrier can lead to food sensitivities, and other issues. Historically, zinc deficiencies were seldom a problem, but the widespread use of PPIs and diets that contain significant amounts of foods that have a relatively high phytate content (especially high-fiber, whole grain diets) has turned it into a modern problem. Not only can a zinc deficiency cause diarrhea, but diarrhea can cause zinc deficiency. So zinc deficiency can become a self-perpetuating problem. Taking a zinc supplement (in the proper balance with copper) is not a primary treatment for MC, but when used as part of a well-thought-out treatment regimen, zinc can definitely help to bring about remission in certain stubborn cases. If zinc supplementation is used, it should be done with about a 15 to 1 ratio of zinc to copper, according to many sources.

Be careful if you take a calcium supplement.

If your doctor has told you to take a calcium supplement, you especially need to make sure that you do not have a magnesium deficiency, and that you actually need a calcium supplement. Very few people actually need a calcium supplement. But most doctors have developed the unfortunate habit of routinely (and inappropriately) promoting the use of calcium supplements in cases where they are not helpful. Most people get more than enough calcium from their diet, even when they are following a restricted diet. The problem is that they either don't absorb it because of a vitamin D deficiency, or they are unable to utilize it because of a magnesium deficiency, or both. If you take a calcium supplement, be sure that your vitamin D level is adequate to allow you to absorb the calcium. And it's always prudent to take magnesium whenever you take a calcium supplement because the calcium to magnesium ratio in your body is closely associated with the risk of colon cancer.

And as we previously discussed, it's also a good practice to take a magnesium supplement whenever vitamin D is supplemented. This will ensure that sufficient magnesium will be available to allow the body to readily convert the vitamin D into the active form as needed by the immune system.

The traditional 2:1 or 3:1 calcium to magnesium ratio recommendations made by many doctors are just flat wrong. They are the result of a translation mistake made years ago (Mercola, 2013, December 08).[169] According to Dr. Carolyn Dean's book *The Magnesium Miracle*, as quoted by Dr. Joseph Mercola, the French researcher Jean Durlach originally stated that one should never ever go beyond a 2:1 calcium to magnesium ratio in one's diet. This was mistakenly interpreted by the medical community to mean that a 2:1 ratio of calcium to magnesium is preferable. It most definitely is not.

A ratio closer to 1:1 is much better for one's health. In fact, Dai et al., (2007) found that not only was increased magnesium intake associated with a lower risk of colorectal cancer, but those who had a certain gene mutation (*1482Ile* allele) were significantly more likely to develop colon cancer as their calcium to magnesium intake ratio increased.[170] The researchers also noted that as magnesium intake increased, the number of polyps in the colon went down.

And as we previously discussed, it's usually helpful to remember that calcium is the only common food ingredient or nutrient known to interfere with the absorption of all forms of iron, whether present in the diet naturally or in supplemental form. Taking a calcium supplement is not nearly as beneficial as most physicians would have us believe.

There are many other vitamins and minerals that impact our health in various ways, but most of them are not a particular problem for microscopic colitis patients, so there's no specific reason to discuss them here. In general though, the vitamin or mineral deficiencies that are discussed in this chapter can have a pronounced effect on our ability to recover from the symptoms of MC. Correcting those particular deficiencies (if they are present) can significantly enhance our immune system's ability to heal our bodies, and help us to recover from the disease. And by comparison, a failure to correct any such deficiencies may possibly prevent or at least postpone the achievement of remission from the symptoms of the disease.

Summary

In this chapter we discovered that magnesium and vitamin D deficiencies are quite commonly associated with MC and a deficiency may seriously interfere with healing. We looked at how much vitamin D we are likely to get from our diet and how much we might get from the sun, and we considered the limitations on these sources. We also discussed the risks associated with supplementation. Furthermore, we discussed how after years of active symptoms, vitamin B deficiency may be a problem. And we discussed how, in some cases, additional deficiencies may develop, such as deficiencies of vitamin A, vitamin B-2, or zinc.

Chapter 4

Methylenetetrahydrofolate Reductase (*MTHFR*) Gene Mutations

MTHFR gene mutations are common and they can cause methylation issues for many people.

In recent years, interest in genes and genomes has been increasing, but the level of understanding that prevails in this area is still rather limited. It's common knowledge that humans normally have 46 chromosomes. An individual inherits 23 chromosomes from her or his mother, and 23 from her or his father. By comparison, wheat has 42 chromosomes.[171] But while wheat may have between 164,000 and 334,000 genes, humans only have about 19,000.[172] Genetics can be tough enough to understand, because of the many possible variations in genes. But this topic becomes downright complicated when we start considering gene mutations.

A mutation is known as a single nucleotide polymorphism (SNP, pronounced snip) and SNPs are located at precise positions along a chromosome where the DNA of different individuals may vary. In general, two alternate options (alleles) are found at any particular SNP. According to the U.S. National Library of Medicine, of the National Institutes of

Health, they occur in human DNA about every 300 nucleotides.[173] A nucleotide is simply a DNA building block that contains the code that defines the genetic options that are available at that particular location in the DNA chain. That implies that there are approximately 10 million SNPs in the human genome. Most of them have little or no effect on our health, but a few have been shown to have major effects on health.

Methylenetetrahydrofolate reductase enzyme modulates the methylation cycle, and this enzyme is encoded by the MTHFR gene. Some basic knowledge about this gene was collected in 2003, when the Human Genome Project was completed. It was discovered that over half the population has one or more mutations of the MTHFR gene (some estimates run as high as 60 %), but so little is known about this whole issue that most people are unaware of just what effects (if any) these gene mutations might have on them.

Because this is such a complex subject and so little is actually known about it in general, it's not surprising that little is known about how this issue might affect MC patients. While researchers have only explored the tip of the iceberg regarding the MTHFR gene, they have sorted out a few associations with various aspects of health, and that allows us to speculate how some of these SNPs might affect a disease such as MC.

In a nutshell, when one's MTHFR gene is healthy, these are the important chemical processes that it initiates.

Note that this only a general overview and if more detailed information is desired, it can be found online at many Internet sources including the stopthethyroidmadness.com webpage.[174] Basically, when everything is working properly, the MTHFR gene initiates a multi-step chemical process known as methylation, which proceeds as follows:

The first step is the production of the MTHFR enzyme. This enzyme breaks down vitamin B-9 (known as folic acid), changing it from 5,10-methylenetetrahydrofolate to 5- methylenetetrahydrofolate. The 5-methylenetetrahydrofolate is then used to convert homocysteine into methionine which is then used by the body for making proteins, using antioxidants, and processing fats.

Methionine can be used to help suppress inflammation and depression symptoms. In the liver, methionine is converted into s-adenosylmethionine (SAM-e). SAM-e is also an anti-inflammatory agent. It is used in the production and subsequent breakdown of neurotransmitters such as serotonin and dopamine; and melatonin, which is a neurotransmitter-like compound. SAM-e is also important in the repair and maintenance of cells.

And here is what can happen when the MTHFR gene is mutated.

When the MTHFR gene is defective, the MTHFR enzyme that's produced performs at only 70 % or 40 % of it's normal capacity, depending on the nature of the gene mutation. This can cause compromised ability of the body to break down and eliminate toxins and heavy metals, and it can lead to a buildup of certain heavy metals. The defective enzyme may not be able to break down and convert folate or folic acid properly, resulting in a buildup of homocysteine, which increases the risk of coronary heart disease and related issues. It can also increase the risk of developing dementia.

Homocysteine conversion to methionine may be compromised, raising the risk of arteriosclerosis, fatty liver disease, anemia, and inflammation. SAM-e production will be decreased, resulting in the likelihood of increased depression symptoms. Because the inactive forms of folate and vitamin B-12 cannot be properly converted into the active forms so that the body can utilize them, the inactive forms of folate and vitamin B-12 may accumulate and this can cause levels to test high. The risk of developing certain cancers may increase. Many diseases have been associated with one or more mutations of the MRHFR gene.

Because genetic mutations can be inherited from both the mother and the father, there are many possible combinations of mutations. The two SNPs that are likely to have the most serious effects on our health are known as C677T and A1298C. Sometimes they are written as just 677 and 1298, because these numbers refer to their location on the gene. If an individual has two copies of either the 677 or the 1298 mutation, it means that that person received one SNP from each parent and he or she is said to be homozygous for that particular mutation. If an individual has one copy of either the 677 or the 1298 mutation from either parent, plus a normal gene that was inherited from the other parent, that person is considered to have a .heterozygous mutation.

23andMe is at the forefront of genetic analysis services that are easily available to the general public.

If you would like to find out which SNPs (if any) you might have, probably the easiest (and most economical) way to find out is to order the test offered by 23andme.[175] The raw data they return after you send in your sample may look like mumbo-jumbo to most people, but the site offers some interpretation services, and various third-party interpretation services are available to provide valuable insight into the meaning of the results that you receive.

Associated websites such as geneticgenie.org offer a free methylation analysis of your raw data to enable you to easily see how you might be affected by your MTHFR gene mutations.[176] Sites such as promethease.-com offer services that will analyze your raw data from 23andME and provide various reports, including some that describe your statistical odds of developing certain diseases as a result of your genetic mutations.[177] And there are many other services offered by other companies that will provide an analysis of your raw 23andMe data. Some reports are free while others are available for a fee. Examples can be found at websites such as livewello.com, codegen.eu, nutrahacker.com, infino.me, enlis.com, and geneknot.com.[178, 179, 180, 181, 182, 183]

Do you know the difference between folate and folic acid?

Even many health professionals will argue that the two terms are interchangeable. But they are not, according to Chris Kressor.[184]

The terms "folate" and "folic acid" are often used interchangeably but they are not one and the same. Folates are members of the B vitamin family (referring to various tetrahydrofolate derivatives) naturally occurring in foods, mainly leafy green vegetables. Folic acid, on the other hand, is a fully oxidized, synthetic compound (pteroylmonoglutamic acid), used in dietary supplements and in food fortification. The important difference to note is that folic acid does not occur naturally.

It's not possible to repair a defective gene, but it's certainly possible to help it to function better.

In the event that you have methylation issues (compromised ability to convert folate and vitamin B-12 into the active forms), you will probably benefit from supplementing with the active forms of folate and vitamin B-12 rather than using the inactive forms. They are 5-methyltetrahydrofolate and methylcobalamin. We have (in the previous chapter) already discussed vitamin B-6 and how it can help to manage histamine levels in the body. For someone who has methylation issues, the proper form to

153

use would be the methyl version of vitamin B-6, which is called pyri-doxal-5-phosphate, or (P5P).

People who have MTHFR mutations often show a high level of copper.

This will usually cause a low level of zinc. The ratio of these two metals is important, but when copper is high, hyperactivity, depression, headaches, acne, poor immune system functioning (resulting in frequent colds), skin sensitivity (easy bruising), low thyroid functioning, or adrenal stress may be a problem. And high copper can frustrate efforts to raise iron levels.

Copper levels can usually be lowered by taking vitamin C, but this should be done slowly, to minimize detoxing symptoms. Taking zinc can also help, but the same precautions regard going slowly should apply.

Over-methylation (also called histapenia) is possible.

Symptoms of over-methylation may include head or neck pain, fatigue, irritability, anxiety, insomnia, depression, paranoia and a tendency to ponder on thoughts. Over-methylated people have elevated levels of serotonin, dopamine, and norepinephrine, and a low histamine level in their blood They tend to be very creative, but they may overreact to common situations in life. Over-methylated individuals also tend to have many food sensitivities, but they are not as likely to react to seasonal allergies.

If you suspect over-methylation, it may help to reduce or stop taking methylating supplements, at least for a while. Some authorities suggest that taking 50 mg time-release capsules of niacin may help if the over-methylation is caused by taking methyl "B" vitamins.

Methylation issues appear to be associated with MC , based on the observation that so many MC patients seem to have histamine-related issues.

Statistically, it's unknown whether MC patients are any more likely than someone in the general population to have MTHFR mutations, but it appears that they may be more likely to experience symptoms because of their level of inflammation due to the disease. Under-methylation (IOW a deficiency of methyfolate) interferes with the production of SAMe, and one of the functions of SAMe is to rid the body of excess histamines. Many MC patients have problems with excess histamine. Experience (and epidemiological data) shows that supplementing with Histame almost never provides any substantial benefits. Histame is sold to replace DAO, and in theory at least, it should be capable of reducing the level of residual (unused/left-over) histamine and therefore prevent histamine levels from reaching problematic levels in the body. Why doesn't it work? Perhaps it doesn't work because the main problem is due to under-methylation. Maybe it doesn't work because SAMe has a much more potent effect on histamine levels than DAO.

Likewise, relatively few MC patients report any significant benefits from taking Gastrocrom. Gastrocrom is sold as a mast cell stabilizer, and it's claimed to help prevent the inappropriate degranulation of mast cells (which results in the dumping of histamine and other pro-inflammatory agents into the bloodstream). Gastrocrom is sometimes prescribed to treat mast cell activation disorder (MCAD), which is known to cause the inappropriate degranulation of mast cells. But again, Gastrocrom is usually reported to not be beneficial in the treatment of MC patients out in the real world. And as is the case with Histame, perhaps this is because SAMe is the primary regulator of histamine levels in the body, and so as a result, products such as Gastrocrom, that do not enhance the production or functionality of SAMe do not have a significant effect on histamine levels in the body.

Summary

Methylation issues are caused by very common genetic mutations of the Methylenetetrahydrofolate reductase (MTHFR) gene, resulting in reduced effectiveness of the MTHFR enzyme. This can lead to many different health problems because when the MTHFR enzyme is defective, the body is unable to properly convert certain vitamins into active forms so that it can use them. Tests may show some of the affected "B" vitamin levels to be either normal or high, but individuals who have methylation issues may still show deficiency symptoms. People who have one or more of these mutations usually benefit from supplementing with the active forms (the methyl forms) of some of the "B" vitamins, instead of taking the regular inactive forms of these vitamins.

Chapter 5

Magnesium Deficiency, Histamine, Gut Bacteria, Inflammation

Histamine is a double-edged sword.

Why is the Mediterranean diet so effective at reducing the risk of heart disease, stroke, diabetes, and other health problems? Probably because the Mediterranean diet contains a lot of magnesium (dailymail.co.uk,. updated 2016, December 8).[185] Why do some studies show vegetarian or vegan diets to provide similar health benefits? Because the only nutrient that a vegan or vegetarian diet contains more of than most conventional diets is magnesium — a lot of magnesium. Magnesium deficiency is the norm in today's world. And that means that any group that is able to avoid magnesium deficiency (by whatever means) can be shown to have a lower risk of many, many health issues, including heart disease, stroke, and diabetes.

Back in chapter 3 we noted that magnesium has been shown to lower CRP levels (King, Mainous, Geesey, & Woolson, 2005). In laboratory rats, a few days of magnesium deficiency tends to create a condition of chronic inflammation (Mazur et al., 2007).[186] This syndrome is characterized by (among other things) leukocyte and macrophage activation, and the release of inflammatory cytokines. The researchers discovered that increasing the magnesium in the cells of the rat decreased the inflammatory response. Mazur et al. (2007) noted that:

> *Moreover, magnesium deficiency induces a systemic stress response by activation of neuro endocrinological pathways. As nervous and immune systems interact bidirectionally, the roles of neuromediators have also been considered. Magnesium deficiency contributes to an exaggerated response to immune stress and oxidative stress is the consequence of the inflammatory response. Inflammation contributes to the pro-atherogenic changes in lipoprotein metabolism, endothelial dysfunction, thrombosis, hypertension and explains the aggravating effect of magnesium deficiency on the development of metabolic syndrome.*

So published research tells us that magnesium deficiency leads to an inflammatory state in the body And this is true independently of any other conditions. By itself, chronic magnesium deficiency is sufficient to establish a state of chronic inflammation. That's a rather profound observation.

Histamine has rather unique properties.

It's an organic nitrogen compound that's released by the immune system in response to both local and systemic immune system provocations. And it can have both local and systemic effects. It's released by mast cells, and by white cells such as basophils and eosinophils to modulate subsequent immune system responses. By doing so, histamine acts both as a physiological function regulator, and a neurotransmitter.

Histamine is responsible for most of the classic allergy symptoms that we experience if we have a pollen allergy or some other type of common allergy. The runny nose, watery eyes, itching, and in severe reactions, the anaphylactic symptoms such as airway restriction and breathing difficulties are caused by the release of histamine. The redness and swelling that develop following a mosquito bite or a wasp sting are due to the release of histamine in the tissues surrounding the bite or sting.

Histamine causes increased permeability of the small blood vessels (capillaries) in the area in order to allow white blood cells to pass from the capillaries into the surrounding tissues to confront any pathogens or toxins that might be present. The inflammation resulting from the histamine and the white cells, along with the fluids from the bloodstream that also flow into the area, cause the redness and swelling.

In the body, histamine is derived from histidine, which is an essential amino acid. Because humans cannot produce histidine, it must be present in the diet. However, certain species of gut bacteria can produce histidine, and it's conceivable that the evolutionary changes that have taken place in our gut bacteria profiles in recent decades due to increased antibiotic use and the expanded use of ingredients and chemicals in processed foods may play a part in the trend toward increasing histamine problems.

We know that histamine is not only vital for immune system functioning, but it's also essential for proper digestion. For example, histamine is released in the stomach to trigger the release of gastric acid by the parietal cells in anticipation of an imminent meal (Håkanson, & Sundler, 1991).[187] However, too much histamine in circulation can cause problems and may be capable of interfering with remission from MC symptoms in some cases.

How is histamine connected with a magnesium deficiency?

Way back in 1987, Nishio, Ishiguro, & Miyao proved that rats fed a magnesium-deficient diet showed significantly increased histamine levels in their urine after 4 days, and the histamine reached a maximum level on day 8.[188] Increased histamine levels could be found in the rats' tissues also, by day 8. When the magnesium deficient group was fed a diet containing a higher magnesium content for 2 days, their histamine (and serum magnesium) levels returned to the same levels as the controls. And additionally, it was noted that by day 8 of a low magnesium diet the diamine oxidase level of the rats was approximately half the level of the controls, which of course compromised the ability of their bodies to purge excess histamine. So the net result of a diet deficient in magnesium is an increase in the histamine level, which is at least partially due to a decreased DAO level.

Is it possible that some MC cases that are resistant to treatment are associated with an undiagnosed magnesium deficiency?

Magnesium deficiency is very common in the general population. In fact, many authorities insist that a majority of the population in developed countries are magnesium-deficient. And magnesium deficiency is even more likely among MC (and other IBD) patients because not only do both the malabsorption problem and the diarrhea associated with the diseases deplete magnesium, but the most common medical treatment used to suppress the inflammation (corticosteroids), also depletes magnesium.

Histidine decarboxylase is the enzyme used by the body to convert histidine into histamine. It's known that a magnesium deficiency increases the activity of histidine decarboxylase, thereby increasing the conversion of histidine into histamine. But a magnesium deficiency can lead to a double whammy in this situation, because it also reduces the activity of DAO (which is normally used by the body to purge excess histamine).

Magnesium Deficiency, Histamine, Gut Bacteria, Inflammation

So with the potential for a significant increase in histamine production, and a reduced ability to remove excessive amounts of histamine from the body, clearly a magnesium deficiency is likely to significantly increase the risk of a histamine buildup that can lead to various problems with the digestive system and elsewhere. And this can occur with or without a shift in the gut bacteria population balance to an increased percentage of histidine-producing bacteria.

If histamine can cause increased permeability of blood vessels, then it doesn't take much of a stretch of the imagination to recognize that it may well also be capable of causing increased permeability of the intestines, because the epithelial lining of both blood vessels and the intestines are quite similar. And because the intestines are specifically designed so that nutrients can pass from the lumen (the interior volume of the intestines) into the blood vessels present in the intestinal walls, for distribution throughout the body, similarity of design of the two interfaces in order to accommodate this vital function would be expected.

Obviously if gut bacteria begin to promote an increase in histidine production concurrent with a magnesium deficiency, this could create the potential for a perfect storm of inflammation due to an inappropriate level of mast cell activity. And the likelihood that this would become a chronic condition means that it would impose a significantly increased risk of triggering and/or perpetuating a microscopic colitis flare. More than several decades ago Watanabe et al. (1981) used mouse embryos to show that mast cells are primarily responsible for histamine levels.[189] They demonstrated this by showing that when mast cells are absent, histidine decarboxylase activity remains low and the histamine level remains low.

Note that because this can happen independently of any white cell-based inflammation that might currently be present, theoretically it can occur even if no white cell infiltration occurs. Or it can occur when a combination of the two modes of inflammation exceed the threshold at which a reaction is triggered. It's possible that there might even be a synergistic effect between the two types of inflammation. And in such a situation, logic dictates that as long as the total sum of the inflammation exceeds the threshold at which a reaction is maintained, remission is not likely to occur.

And because diamine oxidase enzyme requires vitamin B-6 for activation, the deficiency of B vitamins that so commonly occurs over the long term because of the malabsorption problems associated with MC and other IBDs can significantly add to the problem of histamine buildup by preventing DAO from functioning properly. Laboratory experiments have shown that increased vitamin B-6 intake can result in higher DAO activity levels. Whether or not this correlates with improved performance in the real world remains to be seen.

As mentioned earlier in chapter 3, many antibiotics and various other drugs tend to significantly deplete magnesium. And many MC patients point to antibiotics as the cause of their disease. Here is how this cascade of events might unfold to explain why antibiotics can trigger microscopic colitis for so many people:

Antibiotics not only disrupt gut bacteria populations to provide the potential for histidine-producing bacteria to become better established, but many antibiotics also severely deplete magnesium. And as we discussed in the previous section, magnesium deficiency not only increases the activity of histidine decarboxylase, thereby increasing the conversion of histidine into histamine, but it also reduces the activity of diamine oxidase enzyme thereby compromising the ability of the body to purge excess histamine (Nishio, Ishiguro & Miyao, 1987). This sets up an ideal environment for significantly increased mast cell activity and and an inflammatory histamine condition.

Forbes et al. (2008) has demonstrated that when stimulated by inter-leukin-9 (IL-9), increased mast cell activity can cause increased intestinal permeability that leads to food sensitivities.[190] Note that this basically mimics the action of gliadin peptides in wheat gluten, which activate zonulin to cause increased intestinal permeability independent of genet-ics associated with autoimmunity (Drago et al., 2006). In other words, gluten causes increased intestinal permeability in all individuals, not just in those who have a gene associated with celiac disease.

Likewise, the mast cell/histamine conditions de-scribed above appear to provide another mecha-nism that can lead to leaky gut.

This opens the door to a totally independent way for food sensitivities to not only develop, but to be perpetuated, and this has been essentially unexplored by medical researchers. And while this may occur indepen-dently of any genetic limitations, it seems likely that genetics may play a role due to the fact that MC tends to run in families. It's also possible that MC may run in families because of similar environmental associa-tions, rather than genetic links.

But remember that a magnesium deficiency can promote the conversion of histidine to histamine without a gut bacteria population shift. Obvi-ously a much more robust effect would occur if the use of an antibiotic promoted the proliferation of histidine-producing bacteria, but it also appears apparent that this mechanism may be capable of triggering MC independent of an event associated with the use of an antibiotic.

Could mast cell-based inflammation be the primary mode of inflammation associated with MC?

If this theory can be verified, it appears to define a mechanism by which MC can be triggered independently of white cell inflammation. Currently, white cell-based inflammation is generally accepted as the cause of the inflammation. that's associated with the disease. Because lymphocyte-induced inflammation is a diagnostic marker for the disease (LC), this raises an interesting question. "Are there any undiagnosed cases of MC that involve only mast cell-induced inflammation (apart from mastocytic enterocolitis), or do all cases involve white cell-based inflammation?"

The medical description of microscopic colitis attributes the inflammation associated with both lymphocytic colitis and collagenous colitis to increased white cell infiltration into the mucosal and submucosal layers of the epithelial lining of the colon. While thickened collagen bands in the submucosal layer known as the lamina propria are diagnostic markers of collagenous colitis, it's not clear whether the increased thickness is a direct result of inflammation or merely a coincidental marker of CC. But the basic question here is "What if the increased level of white cells is not always the primary source of inflammation?"

If all cases of MC involve lymphocyte-promoted inflammation (by definition), then either all cases initiated by mast cell inflammation soon lead to lymphocytic infiltration, or mast cell-based inflammation (as described above) is concurrent with lymphocyte-based inflammation typically attributed to MC. Otherwise, there is no way that mast cell-based MC cases could be diagnosed under the current diagnostic criteria. Could this be why some symptomatic patients show elevated lymphocyte counts that are not high enough to meet the diagnostic requirement of a minimum of 20 lymphocytes per 100 enterocytes in order to qualify for a diagnosis of LC?

Not only MC, but all other IBDs, and all autoimmune-type diseases may be due to mast cell-based inflammation, rather than lymplocyte-based inflammation.

What if the inflammation that triggers or perpetuates the clinical symptoms associated with MC is caused by too much histamine or inappropriate mast cell activity that results in the release of histamine, cytokines and other proinflammatory immune system agents? We know from published research that mast cells (in the presence of IL-9) can create a condition of increased intestinal permeability (leaky gut) to promote food sensitivities (Forbes et al., 2008). Unfortunately this does not appear to be generally understood by most gastroenterologists because most GI specialists are not trained to recognize the role of mast cells in inflammatory bowel diseases. Rheumatologists often have a much better understanding of mast cell-based inflammation.

But there is compelling epidemiological evidence to suggest that mast cell-induced inflammation sufficient to cause or perpetuate an MC flare may indeed be the driving force behind inflammatory diseases. Perhaps this is why physicians have had so little success in trying to treat autoimmune-type diseases. This could explain why so many cases do not respond to treatment. The most effective treatment found so far is to disable the immune system, putting the patient at the mercy of the pharmaceutical industry, and imposing the risk of developing a fatal infection or cancer. Sadly, instead of treating the cause of the disease, many medical professionals (and patients) choose to simply disable the patients' immune system.

Getting a medical diagnosis of mast cell issues can be tricky.

Because most physicians are not trained to recognize and treat mast cell problems, obtaining an official diagnosis and effective medical treatment for any of the various mast cell disorders will often require traveling in order to locate a qualified doctor or facility. Arguably the most qualified clinicians for dealing with mast cell disorders of various types have been trained at Brigham and Women's Hospital in Boston.[191] Indoctrinated by Dr Mariana Castells, many of these specialists are now located in various parts of the U. S. Dr Castells oversees residents at Brigham and Women's Hospital and Beth Israel Deaconess Medical Center, She also trains students from Harvard Medical School, and fellows in training from the Allergy and Clinical Immunology training programs at Brigham and Women's Hospital, Children's Hospital, and Massachusetts General Hospital.[192]

Diagnosis can be complex, depending on symptoms. About 90 % of cases of mastocytosis involve only the skin and this is referred to as cutaneous mastocytosis. The most severe form of mast cell disorder is systemic mastocytosis, in which case organs other than the skin are involved. Most often, systemic mastocytosis may involve the liver or colon (Scherber & Borate, 2017, October 19).[193] This article gives a reasonably thorough description of the diagnostic process if more detail is desired.

Diets that avoid certain foods referred to as FODMAPs are popular now as a way to treat various digestive issues.

FODMAPs stands for Fermentable Oligosaccharides, Disaccharides, Monosaccharides, and Polyols. It's claimed that FODMAPs are poorly absorbed by some people and because of that they can cause digestive problems. That may well be true, but when I look at a list of the foods that are considered to be high-FODMAP foods, I see a list of high-histamine foods. And when I look at a list of recommended foods (because they are considered to be low-FODMAP foods), I see a list of low-histamine foods. Now not everyone agrees on exactly which foods should be classified as high-histamine and low-histamine. And likewise, there is considerable disagreement between lists that rate the FODMAP status of various foods.

While it's true that not every high-FODMAP food is also a high-histamine food, the FODMAP diet is irrelevant for MC patients who are using diet to control their symptoms. Here's why: If someone is following the diet recommendations for controlling MC, including limiting fiber, sugar, spicy foods, foods that cause their immune system to produce antibodies, and foods that are considered to be high-histamine, then they have no need to worry about high-FODMAP foods because they are already minimizing all of them. Just compare a few lists and you'll see what I mean. So the FODMAP diet is irrelevant for anyone who is already using diet to control their MC.

Summary

Diets that have been proven to reduce cardiovascular disease and other health issues that can lead to increased mortality are high in magnesium content. Magnesium deficiency is very common among the general population. Magnesium deficiency can cause an increase in histamine levels and inflammation. The fact that magnesium deficiency is often associated with MC, and the tendency of a magnesium deficient state to induce a shift in the gut bacteria profile toward higher histidine-producing species could explain how gut bacteria might promote inflammation that leads to the development of, or the perpetuation of, microscopic colitis, in certain cases. Microscopic colitis, together with all other autoimmune-type diseases may be perpetuated by mast cells, possibly as much or more than lymphocytes, in some cases. This is despite the fact that the medical community generally does not consider them to be associated with the disease. High-FODMAP foods are mostly high-fiber and high-histamine foods.

Chapter 6

BAM, SIBO, Low-Dose Naltrexone, GERD, Other Considerations

Bile acid malabsorption (BAM) is a very common cause of chronic diarrhea.

When microscopic colitis fails to respond to treatments that are normally effective, consider a treatment designed to control bile acid malabsorption. Bile acid malabsorption has been shown to be present in 60 % of LC cases and 44 % of CC cases (Ung et al, 2000, Fernandez-Banares et al., 2001).[194, 195] That doesn't mean that the treatment will bring remission in 60 % of LC cases and 44 % of CC cases, but in a few cases that have been unresponsive to other treatments, the diarrhea may stop if a bile acid sequestrant is added to the treatment program.

Based on actual results among members of a microscopic colitis discussion and support forum who tried the treatment, using regular cholestyramine (not the lite version) seems to provide the best results. Be aware that cholestyramine will significantly affect the absorption of nutrients in food and supplements and many medications unless the timing of the dosage is carefully controlled. As a general rule, it should be taken at least two hours after or four hours before eating or taking other medications or vitamin or mineral supplements.

Results suggest that cholestyramine should be considered later in MC treatment programs, rather than as an initial treatment.

Informally comparing the results of those who tried cholestyramine early in their treatment program with the results of those who tried it later in their treatment, it appears that in most cases, success rates have been significantly higher for those MC patients who have used cholestyramine after they have been treating the disease for more than a year, but have been unsuccessful in completely stopping the diarrhea.

This is almost surely because the diet changes need to be made and the inflammation from food sensitivities needs to be suppressed before the bile acid sequestrant is likely to be effective. In cases of BAM without a diagnosis of MC, the diet changes might not be necessary. But with MC, early on, the reaction due to inflammation from food sensitivities is likely to overwhelm the medication's ability to stop the diarrhea by sequestering the bile acids in most cases. After the inflammation has been suppressed by diet changes, so that the principal remaining issue is the BAM, then the cholestyramine should be more effective.

Gastroenterologists seem to prefer trying a cholestyramine treatment early on simply because of the prevalence of BAM relative to MC. But BAM is not the primary cause of diarrhea in the early stages of MC. The diarrhea is primarily due to the intestinal inflammation. BAM may be present early on, but that may be overshadowed by the secretory diarrhea associated with MC. After the lymphocyte levels have been suppressed by diet changes, then if remission is still elusive, it might be time to consider BAM as the possible cause of the remaining diarrhea. The key to successfully bringing remission to MC patients in many cases may lie in finding the optimum dose. That, of course, must be done by trial and error.

Cholestyramine also has other uses for MC patients.

It can be used to bind various toxins and remove them from the body. For example, MC patients sometimes develop Clostridium difficile infections. Colestyramine can be used by patients who have a C. difficile infection to absorb toxins A and B (produced by the bacteria), and thereby reduce the diarrhea and the other symptoms that these toxins usually cause. However, cholestyramine does not treat a C. difficile infection, so it must be used used together with vancomycin, or some other appropriate antibiotic in order to control the infection. And because the cholestyramine can decrease the effectiveness of many medications, including antibiotics, the Vancomycin (or other antibiotic) should be taken at least one or two hours before or 4–6 hours after taking the cholestyramine

Recycling of bile acids appears to be controlled by cortisol.

Experimenting with specially-altered mice (mice that had no glucocorticoid receptors in their livers), Rose et al. (2011) found that compared with normal mice, they lost weight on the same diet because their ability to digest fat was compromised.[196] They weren't able to normally recycle bile acids and they developed gallstones.

An adequate supply of bile is stored in the gallbladder. When the body becomes hungry, it releases cortisol (which is a glucocorticoid). Cortisol is a hormone and it attaches to the glucocorticoid receptors in the liver and the liver responds by producing bile and storing it in the gallbladder, in anticipation of the next meal. When the meal is actually eaten, bile is released through the common bile duct into the small intestine to emulsify the fat in the food. Additionally, lipase from the pancreas is added to the bile in the common bile duct to further digest the fat in the small intestine.

Normally, the body recycles about 90–95 % of the bile that's released into the small intestine. It's reabsorbed in the terminal ileum (the last section of the small intestine). If it's not reabsorbed, and too much of it passes into the colon, it may cause diarrhea. This is the essence of bile acid malabsorption.

But in addition, if bile acids are not adequately reabsorbed, the liver may soon be unable to maintain a normal level of bile in the gallbladder because without the recycling, it simply cannot produce enough bile. And the body's ability to digest fat will be limited, leading to weight loss. Thus the researchers were able to prove that cortisol controls the recycling of bile acids.

Rose et al. (2011) also discovered that this effect apparently also applies to humans. Cortisol is normally produced by the adrenal glands. When people have a rare disorder called Addison's disease, their immune system attacks their adrenal glands and their ability to produce normal amounts of cortisol is disrupted. The researchers found that when they examined blood samples of Addison's disease patients taken before and after eating, bile acid recycling was also compromised, similar to the mice that had no glucocorticoid receptors in their livers. So apparently cortisol also controls bile acid recycling in humans.

This appears to have interesting implications for MC patients.

This suggests that MC patients who tend to lose weight during a flare may be short of cortisol. And too much undigested fat in the colon can cause diarrhea. This also might suggest that such individuals may not be able to properly recycle bile acids and may therefore possibly be more likely to respond to cholestyramine treatment than those who do not usually lose weight during an MC flare. There is no published medical research to confirm this, therefore, this is strictly a speculative observation. It may have merit, but there is no medical proof.

The discovery that cortisol controls bile acid recycling would surely have implications for patients taking a corticosteroid to treat MC.

Products such as budesonide (Entocort or Uceris) obviously must be capable of boosting bile acid absorption, since budesonide is an anti-inflammatory corticosteroid with potent glucocorticoid activity. So perhaps it is this capability of improving bile acid absorption that is responsible for stopping the diarrhea in only one or two days in certain cases. Perhaps this explains why some patients who take budesonide are more likely to gain weight as a side effect of the drug.

Here are some tips regarding taking budesonide for optimum effectiveness during recovery.

The way that most gastroenterologists prescribe the use of budesonide to treat MC usually results in a relapse rate of up to 82 % when the treatment is ended (Park, Cave, & Marshall, 2015).[197] Eliminating all food sensitivities from the diet is critical for success. If budesonide is used in addition to diet changes for treating MC, then tapering the dose as the treatment is ended is crucial, and doing it properly can be confusing. Here are some guidelines. In this situation, the purpose of the budesonide is simply to mask the symptoms while the diet heals the intestines. But if ending the treatment causes the diarrhea to return, then three possibilities exist:

1. The dose is being tapered too soon — the diet changes have not had sufficient time for enough healing to take place.

2. The diet is either cross-contaminated by a known food sensitivity or contaminated by an unrecognized food sensitivity.

3. A combination of the first two possibilities exists.

The only reason for taking budesonide is to mask the symptoms . It only treats the symptoms, not the root cause of the symptoms. The root cause of the symptoms is intestinal inflammation. While budesonide does indeed help to suppress inflammation, it cannot stop the inflammation from being regenerated with each meal — only diet changes can do that. So the fact remains that Budesonide doesn't address the root cause of the problem.

But taking budesonide can mask the symptoms of food sensitivities in some cases. This can make fine tuning one's recovery diet rather tricky. Because of that issue, some people prefer to not take budesonide while they are recovering on an elimination diet. As was discussed in the first edition of *Microscopic Colitis*, corticosteroids do not speed up healing — published research shows that they slow down the healing rate somewhat. But they can make life much more pleasant during recovery, even though they may do so at the expense of slightly extending healing time. And as noted above, if the cause of continued diarrhea is bile acid malabsorption, then budesonide may be an aid to recovery in that respect.

The time to reach remission can vary by a great deal, but it usually ranges from three to six months. For that reason, most people who successfully use budesonide to mask the symptoms while they are healing the intestinal damage by following a restricted diet, begin to slowly taper the dose of budesonide after about three (or more) months at full dose (unless constipation prompts them to reduce the dose sooner), and they complete the taper to end the treatment about three months (or more) later, for a full treatment regimen of about six months or longer.

Ideally, one should be able to remain relatively diarrhea-free, while still being able to detect food sensitivities by taking just enough budesonide to prevent diarrhea, but only taking enough to prevent diarrhea when all of one's food sensitivities are avoided. It can be a relatively fine distinction. The proper way (or at least the optimum way) to taper budesonide seems to be to reduce the dose as soon as one notices signs of constipation, rather than reducing the dose based on a rigid time schedule. Following a set time schedule rarely works well, because there is so much variation in the way that many patients respond to budesonide.

It has been suggested that fibroblast growth factor 19 (FGF19) might be useful for treating bile acid problems.

Not only is bile acid normally reabsorbed in the terminal ileum but this action triggers the production of FGF19, a hormone that's produced in the terminal ileum. Normally, blood levels of FGF19 increase following a meal and FGF19 hormone regulates the production of bile in the liver according to the needs of the digestive system (Lundåsen, Gälman, Angelin & Rudling, 2006).[198] But the inflammation associated with active Crohn's disease has been shown to reduce the blood level of this hormone (Nolan et al., 2015).[199] Surgical shortening of the ileum also results in reduced FGF19 production. Walters (2014) discussed how monkeys without FDF19 developed severe diarrhea.[200] All of which has prompted Walters and Appleby, (2015) to demonstrate that a similar protein, M70 can be injected to produce the same effects as FGF19, thereby providing a possible bile acid malabsorption treatment option.[201] How well this might work for MC patients, remains to be seen.

Here's why bile acid sequestrants may not be such a great choice for treating MC.

Bile acid sequestrants were developed to lower cholesterol, not to treat MC. When cholestyramine or a similar product is taken, bile acids are tied up by the drug and purged (because they will remain in the stool and end up in the toilet). They cannot be recycled, so bile acid absorption will decrease dramatically. By contrast, if budesonide is taken to treat MC, the cortisol boost means that bile acid absorption will increase, which is the opposite effect of a bile acid sequestrant. This results in improved fat absorption, allowing patients to gain weight, rather than lose weight.

The bottom line is that bile acid sequestrants such as cholestyramine may seem like a good idea, but the fact that their use results in the wholesale loss of bile acids and the fat that they were put there to digest in the first place, means that their actual usefulness is significantly compromised unless the goal is to lose weight. Using bile acid sequestrants tends to waste fat, and many MC patients can ill afford to lose the fat in their diet.

Correcting the problem of fat and bile acid malabsorption is definitely a useful goal for treating MC. But trying to correct the problem by flushing bile acids and fat down the toilet seems to be a rather poor solution. Patients need those bile acids and fat for their health. Therefore, if one is going to use a drug to treat the disease, budesonide appears to be a much more practical choice than cholestyramine.

But all medications have undesirable side effects. Budesonide is far less likely to suppress the functioning of the adrenals than the other corticosteroids, but eventually, if used long enough, it will begin to suppress adrenal function. And of course that will reduce cortisol production which will promote reduced bile acid recycling and reduced fat absorption. Perhaps this is why many patients find that budesonide is less effective as time passes, and it may eventually stop working for them.

Small intestinal bacterial overgrowth (SIBO)

SIBO is defined as an abnormally high number of bacteria in the small intestine (Dukowicz, Lacy, & Levine, 2007).[202] It's frequently claimed to be the cause of chronic diarrhea and malabsorption, particularly by naturopathic practitioners. But in the real world, a shift in the balance among bacterial species is frequently considered to be SIBO. The reality is that species of bacteria and balances among those species in our intestines tend to change as our diet is changed and as our digestive abilities changes during the course of the disease.

Poor digestion leads to increases in population levels of certain opportunistic species that can benefit from the fermentation of partially-digested food. As the gut heals, and digestion improves, those species are "starved out" and replaced by some of the species of bacteria that were there originally. Likewise, as we change our diet to eat more protein and less carbohydrates, bacterial species that thrive on the altered diet tend to crowd out species that can't compete when fed that particular food. And as we heal, and gradually go back to eating some of the foods that were originally cut out of our diet, the bacterial balance among the various species of gut bacteria will shift again, to reflect the new diet.

Naturopaths often recommend testing for SIBO. And of course the testing almost always finds "SIBO" in patients with active microscopic colitis because SIBO has been found to be associated with many diseases.[203] So they recommend treating the "SIBO". But just because "SIBO" happens to be associated with a disease does not mean that it caused the disease. Fire trucks can be found near fires, but they are virtually never the cause of the fire. Is it really SIBO, or just a natural shift in the balances among the various bacterial species in response to diet changes or to loss of digestive efficiency as a result of the disease?

Digestive diseases create opportunities for bacteria, so they can hardly be blamed for for taking advantage of the situation. Logic suggests that SIBO is not the likely cause of all of the diseases attributed to it. It's much more likely that those diseases cause SIBO. Virtually every one of the diseases associated with SIBO is related to, or caused by a digestive system disorder. Digestive diseases naturally tend to cause poor digestion and poor digestion causes changes in gut bacteria populations as opportunistic bacteria take advantage of undigested or poorly-digested food to establish colonies that thrive under such conditions. So it's much more likely that digestive system problems cause SIBO than SIBO causes digestive system diseases. Consequently, there's little point in treating SIBO because that is simply treating a symptom— it's not treating the cause of the symptom. When the cause of the symptom is resolved, then the symptom will automatically disappear.

As the inflammation decreases, in response to proper diet changes, bacterial balances tend to realign to a more normal pattern in most patients, regardless of whether or not "SIBO" is treated. The point is, what may be interpreted as SIBO will usually be corrected automatically without any intervention, as the microscopic colitis is brought under control by stopping the inflammation with diet changes that avoid the inflammatory foods.

So in most cases, the "SIBO" tends to be a symptom of MC, rather than the MC being a symptom of SIBO. Except for truly pathogenic populations of certain species, treating a gut bacteria balance shift is usually pointless, because after the treatment, the balance among the various species populating the intestines is going to be determined by diet and the effectiveness of the digestive system at that point in time. So the population balance will tend to sort out according to those criteria after a few weeks. That said, if a true infection exists, it should be treated. Normally however, treating "SIBO" associated with MC appears to be a waste of time and money for many patients.

Low dose naltrexone (LDN) has been used as an alternative treatment for many autoimmune diseases.

Originally used primarily to manage a dependency on alcohol or opioid-based drugs, naltrexone in very low doses is currently the darling of those seeking alternative treatments for many autoimmune diseases. The idea behind low dose naltrexone is to reset the immune system to try to "kick" it out of a regular pattern of reactions against an antigen, thus stopping autoimmune type reactions. A quick review of the literature shows that it seems to show promise as a treatment for pain and symptom severity for many diseases (Younger, Parkitny, & McLain, 2014).[204] But is it effective for treating microscopic colitis?

To date many people have tried to use LDN to treat many diseases, including microscopic colitis. Have they been successful? With many diseases, indications are that yes, LDN treatments have often been successful at bringing relief of symptoms. But with MC, LDN treatment seems to be successful at relieving symptoms only when the patient has other autoimmune issues that have been preventing remission from MC.

Reports of the successful use of LDN for treating MC that can be authenticated are lacking. There are virtually no valid published medical research articles in this area in the literature. In other words, treating MC with LDN has not been proven to be generally successful. However, no one has conclusively proven that it cannot be used to treat MC, either. It's possible that it can be used to treat other issues (other autoimmune issues) that have been preventing remission of MC symptoms, in order to allow MC to go into remission. For example, in the case of type

1 diabetes patients who have MC, there have been case reports of successfully resolving MC symptoms by using LDN. This issue is in desperate need of medical research studies to prove or disprove the efficacy of LDN for treating MC.

Would it help to take L-glutamine?

Body builders take L-glutamine in order to help build muscles. L-glutamine is believed to help heal injured muscle tissue. Some people believe that because the intestines are primarily comprised of muscle tissue, L-glutamine should help heal them also. But here's why that reasoning may be faulty:

Muscle tissue in the intestines begins with the muscularis mucosae, which is the third (looking from the inside out) layer of the mucosa, and of course there is smooth muscle below that, in the walls of the intestines. With Crohn's disease and ulcerative colitis, damage (in the form of physical lesions) can occur to any and all layers of the intestinal walls from the epithelium all the way out to the serosa (the outermost layer). But with MC, intestinal damage only involves the top 2 (innermost) layers, the epithelium and the lamina propria. And it's not physical damage of the type that lesions would cause — it's inflammatory damage. Neither the epithelium nor the lamina propria contain any muscle tissue. Because of that, it's unlikely that L-glutamine would speed up intestinal healing for MC patients. It might help healing in the case of Crohn's disease and ulcerative colitis. It's not impossible that it might help heal the gut for MC patients, but if it does, it does so by some unknown mechanism, not by the claims typically made for it.

Gastroesophageal reflux disease (GERD) is somewhat commonly associated with MC

Any digestive system issues that typically result in poor digestion predispose patients to the possible development of acid reflux, heartburn, and gas. Eventually those issues are likely to lead to the development of GERD. And since the medication most likely to be prescribed to treat GERD is a proton pump inhibitor (PPI), and PPIs are well known for triggering MC, this rapidly becomes a self-perpetuating problem. PPIs tend to cause a dependency after a couple of weeks of use. And because they are a trigger for MC, their use must be stopped, not only because remission cannot be achieved as long as they are being used, but for general health reasons as well. They have been shown to cause the very symptom that they are prescribed to treat. Research published by Reimer, Sondergaard, Hilsted, and Bytzer (2009) and McColl and Gillen, (2009) proves that after eight weeks of using a PPI, even healthy subjects produce excessive stomach acid.[205, 206]

Furthermore the FDA has mandated the addition of "black box" warnings on the label to advise users that the use of PPIs carries an increased risk of causing such problems as kidney damage, Alzheimer's , and other forms of age-related dementia (Sampathkumar, Ramalingam, Prabakar, & Abraham, 2013, Fallahzadeh, Borhani Haghighi, & Namazi, 2010, Haenisch et al., 2015).[207, 208, 209] And we know from experience and case studies that using a PPI carries an increased risk of developing osteoporosis, bacterial infections (especially C. diff), and problems with decreased digestive abilities.

The idea that excess stomach acidity is so widespread among the general population that it needs to be treated is preposterous in the first place. Younger people rarely have problems with too much stomach acidity, and the ability to produce gastric acid in sufficient quantities for good digestion normally declines as we age — it almost never increases. So why do physicians feel the need to prescribe PPIs for so many of their patients — especially when PPIs have so many negative health risks?

Over the years, many, many patients have regretted following their doctor's advice to take a PPI. After medium to long-term use, when the time comes to stop using a PPI, most people discover that they have sig-nificantly worse health issues because of taking the drug than they had before they started taking it. When trying to wean off the use of a PPI, the rebound acid hypersecretion (RAHS) problem is well known, be-cause it makes discontinuing the use of the drug very difficult. It makes the symptoms much worse than they were before the treatment was started because the acid production increases dramatically as the drug is withdrawn.

Many people will find it necessary to use an H2 blocker to lower the acidity in the stomach while withdrawing from PPI use. PPIs have some efficacy for about three days, even though they are normally taken daily. H2 blockers are only effective for a few hours, so they will need to be taken much more frequently.

The backside (the stomach side) acidity to which the lower esophageal sphincter (LES) is exposed determines the clenching strength of the LES. The higher the acidity, the tighter it normally clinches. By lowering the acidity, PPIs lower the clenching strength of the LES. And over the long term, this weakens the LES (the LES is a muscle and when we don't use muscles, they tend to become weaker).

But the patient never notices this weakening as long as she or he is tak-ing a PPI because the PPI deactivates the acidity so effectively that the stomach contents don't burn the esophagus when they are refluxed. When PPIs are discontinued, it doesn't take long before the burning be-comes painfully obvious. Thus the need for an H2 blocker.

Stopping a PPI treatment cold turkey is rarely an option if they have been used for a long period of time. It's more practical to step down the dose (by skipping the PPI treatment on alternate days, then skipping two days, and so fourth) in order to wean off the PPI, and replacing the PPI with H2 blockers as needed to lower the stomach acidity. It's much easier to eventually wean off an H2 blocker because they don't cause the acid-rebound problem created by all PPIs.

The common H2 blockers are:

- Famotidine (Pepcid AC, Pepcid Oral)
- Cimetidine (Tagamet, Tagamet HB)
- Ranitidine (Zantac, Zantac 75, Zantac Efferdose, Zantac injection, and Zantac Syrup)
- Nizatidine Capsules (Axid AR, Axid Capsules, Nizatidine Capsules)

One option to consider is taking a vitamin D supplement, or increasing the dose if vitamin D is already being taken. Anecdotal evidence exists to suggest that taking 5,000–10,000 IU of vitamin D daily while trying to wean off a PPI may help to reduce GERD symptoms (Cannell, (2011, September 07, Rathod, 2017, September 18).[210, 211] The reason why vitamin D can help in this situation is probably because (as we discussed previously) vitamin D regulates the absorption of calcium. Calcium (usually in the form of calcium carbonate) has a long history of use as an antacid providing a good remedy for heartburn, acid indigestion and similar issues. Enhancing the absorption of calcium by taking vitamin D allows our body to absorb the calcium already in our diet to provide the benefits of taking an antacid without actually taking one.

If doses of more than 5,000 IU of vitamin D are taken regularly, one's blood level of vitamin D should be checked after a few months to make sure that it isn't getting up over the optimum level of 40 to 80 ng/ml (100 to 200 mmol/l). Exceeding the optimum level is not a major problem, but care should be taken to see that it doesn't exceed what is considered to the overdose level of about 150 ng/ml (375 nmol), as having a 25(OH)D level in that range can cause digestive upset.

Taking a magnesium supplement will usually also be beneficial — not only because magnesium helps to activate vitamin D, but because a magnesium deficiency may make it easier for GERD to develop. This is because a magnesium deficiency will usually cause muscle weakness and spasming, and both the lower esophageal sphincter at the bottom of the esophagus and the pyloric sphincter at the bottom of the stomach are muscles. Helping those muscles to relax and stop spasming will help the LES to remain more tightly clinched, and will help the pyloric sphincter to allow the stomach to empty in a more timely manner. When the stomach doesn't empty as soon as it should, gas pressure can build up to cause the stomach contents to backflow, and of course that results in acid reflux into the esophagus.

A low-carb diet can be very beneficial as a way to minimize or resolve acid reflux or heartburn symptoms.[212] Alternative medicine practitioners often resolve reflux and heartburn problems of their patients by recommending a low-carb diet.

Does a melatonin deficiency cause GERD or does GERD cause a melatonin deficiency?

Kandil, Mousa, El-Gendy, & Abbas (2010) have shown that melatonin is effective for treating GERD and therefore it may be helpful when weaning off a PPI.[213] The researchers found that baseline evaluations of subjects enrolled in their study showed that when compared with controls (who did not have GERD) the subjects who did have GERD had significantly lower levels of melatonin.

The report suggested that melatonin might be useful for treating GERD. It showed that 3 mg of melatonin taken at bedtime was often effective for preventing GERD.

The association of the deficiency of melatonin with GERD had been previously found by Klupińska et al. (2006).[214] In this paper the researchers noted that:

> The findings of this study support the notion that melatonin exerts beneficial influences on the upper digestive tract. It is likely that high or relatively correct secretion of melatonin is sufficient to prevent peptic changes in esophageal and duodenal mucosa. (p. 1)

Unfortunately, additional research to show that melatonin is useful for treating GERD is not very likely due to the fact that most medical research today is financed by the major pharmaceutical companies. No pharmaceutical company is likely to spend any money proving that something as cheap as melatonin is useful for treating GERD when they are all making billions of dollars by promoting the use of PPIs to treat the problem.

To minimize the risk of having acid reflux and to make weaning off a PPI easier, there are a number of guidelines that should be followed. Avoiding certain foods can help significantly. As we discussed previously, minimizing carbohydrates in the diet is a good first step. Such foods as chocolate, alcohol, coffee, tomatoes (or other sources of citric a id), and peppermint are well known for causing acid reflux or making it worse.

Reflux problems are usually more severe during the night because of the recumbent position while sleeping. While some foods might not cause any reflux problems during the daytime, avoiding them becomes especially important at night, and as a general rule they should be totally avoided during the period beginning several hours before bedtime.

Anyone with reflux problems should always sleep on their back or on their left side, never on their right side or any position that might put pressure on the stomach. This is because the lower esophageal sphincter is lower than parts of the stomach when someone lies on their right side. In that position, if the LES does not remain tightly clinched at all times, the contents of the stomach will surely backflow into the esophagus.

It's important to prevent this from happening. It's more likely to happen if an antacid or H2 blocker (or especially a PPI) is being used. The head of the bed can even be elevated slightly (by placing bricks or other blocks under the legs, for example) to further assist in preventing reflux.

If you need help, here are some suggestions for using an H2 blocker to help wean off a PPI.[215]

- Reduce the dosage of the PPI by approximately 25–50 % per week. The slower the dose is tapered, the less likely that the acid rebound effect will be a problem.

- First reduce the amount taken and then reduce how often it is taken by taking it every other day. The increasing acidity will probably begin to cause symptoms at some point. If it doesn't, great, you're home free.

- If it causes heartburn symptoms, take an H2 blocker. Antacids can also be used to supplement the effect of the H2 blocker if needed.

- Continue to reduce the dose of the PPI until the dose is low enough to discontinue it.

- After you have been off the PPI for a week, you should be able to start reducing the dose of the H2 blocker. Weaning off the H2 blocker should be easier than getting off the PPI.

- Antacids (or an H2 blocker) can be used, as needed, if occasional heartburn is a problem in the future.

Behold the power of placebos.

And as a last thought, consider the power of placebos. Placebos are pills that contain no medications. A CBS TV show presented the details of a research project in which IBS patients were treated with a placebo.[216] Surprisingly, the placebo treatment had a 60 % success rate at relieving symptoms, which is about as good as can be expected from many medications under similar circumstances. The study was done at Boston's Beth Israel Deaconess Medical Center.

But what really makes this project fascinating is the fact that the subjects in the study were told that they were receiving placebos. And the project still had a 60 % success rate. Why? Obviously the mind has powers that we don't completely understand. The mind can sometimes be used to force the body to accept things that it would not otherwise accept.

No one is suggesting that anyone should try to treat MC with placebos, but on the other hand, this proves that a positive attitude can go a long way — especially when treating a miserable digestive-system disease. This disease can be tough to treat, and many treatments have been met with failure.

The point is that despite the depressing ambiance of the disease, a positive attitude will almost surely get you to remission faster than a negative attitude. Among the many benefits of having a positive attitude is the likelihood that you will be totally diligent in all your efforts, and diligence can be crucial to success.

This isn't just wishful thinking. The healing powers of positive thinking have been discussed by many authors, as attested to by a *Psychology Today* article by Dr. Lissa Rankin (2011, December 27).[217] While positive thinking may not rescue a terminally ill patient, when used in the early stages of a disease and for one's health in general, attitude can definitely make a difference.

Summary

As many as 60 % of LC cases and 44 % or CC cases have been shown to be associated with bile acid malabsorption. This suggests that cholestyramine may be very useful for treating MC.

In reality, however, cholestyramine does not seem to have a high success rate for treating MC and despite the fact that it is considered to be a relatively safe treatment, it has some rather undesirable side effects. It works by wasting bile acids instead of recycling them, and this leaves the body unable to absorb fat, which is a major disadvantage for many MC patients, unless they need to lose weight.

SIBO is claimed to be a major cause of digestive system upset, but it appears that SIBO is usually a consequence of MC rather than a cause. Treating it usually does not eliminate the problem for more than a few weeks. SIBO normally resolves automatically as the MC is brought under control.

Low-dose naltrexone seems to be helpful for reducing symptoms of many autoimmune diseases. So far however, it hasn't been shown to be useful for controlling the symptoms of MC, unless the case in question is refractive to treatment because of some other AI disease that can be successfully treated by LDN.

GERD is very commonly associated with MC because of the poor digestion usually caused by the disease. Vitamin D, magnesium, and avoiding certain foods that promote reflux can be used to help control or prevent it.

Attitude is important. It determines how we perceive ourselves in relation to the rest of the world. Recovery from MC and various other diseases may happen sooner when a positive attitude is maintained.

Chapter 7

Depression, Inflammation, and Stress Associated with MC

Many MC patients can trace the origins of their disease to a particularly stressful event.

Many, many cases of MC have resulted from the severe stress associated with the loss of a loved one, whether the loss be a mate, a family member, a close friend, or a four-legged companion. Case studies show that such losses also tend to trigger relapses for many people, even when they have been in stable remission for years. In most cases, severe stress seems to be capable of defeating even the best of treatment or maintenance programs.

Many MC patients are depressed. MC is a depressing disease. And some cases of MC have apparently been triggered by the use of antidepressant medications. In a small double-blind cross-over study, Peters, Biesiekierski, Yelland, Muir, and Gibson (2014) demonstrated that people who have non-celiac gluten sensitivity develop symptoms of depression when exposed to gluten.[218] Gluten had previously been shown to cause major depression symptoms for people who have celiac disease (Carta et al., 2002).[219]

Back in 2001, Kurina, Goldacre, Yeates, and Gill (2001) proved that IBD patients tend to have higher-than-normal rates of depression and anxiety.[220] In fact, they showed that the symptoms can exist for up to a year before diagnosis of an IBD. In ulcerative colitis patients (but not Crohn's disease), a history of depression could be found for five or more years in advance of the diagnosis of the IBD. It's difficult not to believe that the depression might have contributed to the eventual diagnosis in at least some of those cases.

Some authorities believe that depression is a disease.

And a good case can be made that depression is due to the production of cytokines (Smith, 1997).[221] Smith summarizes the case eloquently:

> There is considerable immunological evidence supporting immune activation and cytokine secretion as important processes underlying depression. First, cytokines given chronically to human volunteers can produced (sic) all the symptoms necessary for the diagnosis of depression. Second, depressed patients secrete more cytokine than normal controls. The level of cytokine secretion is closely linked with the severity of the depression. Third, depressed patients have activated immune systems. The most severely depressed patients have the most activated immune systems. Furthermore, immune activation is the cause of the concurrent immunosuppression reported with depression.

But other authorities believe that depression is a symptom, rather than a disease.

Depression can be shown to be a result of inflammation, so many people believe that it's a symptom (of inflammation).[222] They believe that all disease is associated with inflammation, and therefore depression is associated with virtually all diseases. According to Berk et al. (2013) this association has been demonstrated for at least the following issues:[223]

- Stress and trauma
- Diet
- Exercise
- Obesity
- Smoking
- Gut permeability, the microbiome, and the TLR-IV pathway
- Atopic disorders (hyperallergic disorders)
- Dental cares and peridontal diseases
- Sleep
- Vitamin D
- Psychiatric disorders

But despite all the medical evidence that depression is caused by inflammation, it is still treated as a chemical imbalance by the medical community.

It's still treated by using medications that regulate chemical hormones such as serotonin, norepinephrine, and dopamine — medications that we refer to as antidepressants. Why do medical professionals still prefer to use this obsolete approach to treat depression twenty or thirty years after research was published to show that inflammation is the problem, not chemical imbalance? They apparently do so because pharmaceutical companies are making so much money out of this that they have managed to "outshout" researchers with their campaigns to convince the public and practicing physicians that antidepressants work (even though plenty of evidence exists to show that they are barely better than placebos (Kirsch, 2014; Begley, 2010, January 28).[224, 225] It could be argued that clinicians are reluctant to change because they don't really understand depression, so it's not surprising that they also don't understand how to properly treat it.

Alzheimer's, arthritis, cancer, and cardiovascular disease all have a common cause — inflammation.

Inflammation is the body's response to stress. Inflammation can be caused by many things, including, but not limited to (Inflammation: The Real Cause of All Disease and How to Reduce and Prevent It, n.d.):[226]

- Chronic bacterial, viral, or fungal infections of the bloodstream or organs in the digestive system
- Food allergies or food sensitivities
- SIBO or other forms of gut microbiota dysbiosis
- Environmental toxins and allergens (such as molds, fungus, pollen, or metals such as mercury, lead, and cadmium
- Diet or lifestyle issues
- Stress

Inflammation can result in clinical symptoms such as:

- Wrinkles and other visible signs of aging
- Increased susceptibility to bacterial, fungal, and viral infections
- Acid reflux or gastroesophageal reflux disease (GERD)
- Some types of cancer
- Eczema, psoriasis, acne and other skin disorders
- Arthritis or other joint issues
- Bronchitis and chronic sinusitis
- Chronic pain
- Type 2 Diabetes
- Hypertension
- Osteoporosis

- Cardiovascular disease
- Candidiasis (yeast overgrowth)
- Recurring urinary tract infections

Whether stress is due to physical, chemical, mental, or emotional duress, the effect is typically the same — inflammation.

Researchers have proven the effects of social stress by doing an experiment with mice (Powell et al., 2013).[227] They showed that a stressful social setting resulted in the up-regulation (activation) of 3,000 genes in the stressed mice and 1,142 of those genes contributed to increasing the level of inflammation associated with the immune system. Researchers have found similar responses to stress in humans (Huffington Post, 2013, November 11).[228]

Stress affects every part of the body (News-Medical Life Sciences, 2008, January 9).[229] Inherited from our evolutionary past, the stress response results in the release of hormones (from our adrenal glands) such as epinephrine (adrenaline), norepinephrine, and cortisol. These hormones cause an increase in our heart rate, our breathing, and glucose in our blood so that the fuel is available for the fight-or-flight situation that is anticipated by the body. This requires a lot of energy, so the digestive system, the reproductive system, growth (in young people), and some functions of the immune system are either shut down or significantly slowed down.

When such situations pass quickly, cortisol levels return to near-normal within about an hour, and so the digestive system and all the other affected systems soon resume normal functioning. Food that was only partially-digested when the crisis occurred may spoil and need to be purged, but this is normally just a passing problem. If the problem becomes chronic, due to a continuing stressful situation, proper digestion can be more significantly compromised. If this continues for an extended period, the digestive environment becomes more suitable for the development of microscopic colitis or other digestive system issues.

Even trying to explain the disease to friends, family members, co-workers or neighbors in a way that they will understand is almost always stressful.

Most people don't understand chronic food sensitivity issues. And that's not surprising because as we will learn in the next chapter, even most medical professionals don't understand them. A typical response from most people is usually something such as, "But you don't look sick", or "You can't believe everything you read on the Internet", or "Just try a little of this desert — a little can't hurt".

So how can we explain it in a way that they will understand what we are dealing with? It might be helpful to point out that for many microscopic colitis patients, having MC is a lot like having the flu — permanently. If a patient can't figure out what is causing the inflammation, he or she may continue to react forever, with flu-like symptoms. It's kind of like a pollen allergy, but it affects the digestive system instead of the respiratory system. The only way to stop it is to totally avoid the foods or medications that are causing it. That means permanent lifestyle changes.

Summary
Stress, inflammation, and depression are all linked, and they surely contribute to the development of many diseases, especially autoimmune diseases. The mainstream medical community appears to misunderstand this association and as a result, depression, which has been shown to be a symptom of the stress caused by untreated gluten sensitivity, is

mistakenly treated as a chemical imbalance in the body. When this condition is improperly treated, the stage is set for the development of various autoimmune diseases, including inflammatory bowel disease.

Chapter 8

Medical Diagnostic and Treatment Issues That Should Be Corrected

The issues discussed in this chapter and the suggested modifications are based strictly on the opinions of the author, and nothing more.

There are many practices or policies that are currently being followed by the medical community that are either not providing the benefits in patient care claimed, or they are actually causing harm. Correcting these issues would provide substantial benefits in patient care.

In far too many cases, MC appears to be an iatrogenic disease — a consequence of a prior medical treatment. Many cases appear to be the result of drugs that were prescribed to treat other issues. And in most of those situations, other treatment options were available that could have significantly reduced the risk of causing an inflammatory bowel disease.

Perhaps the easiest way to treat MC is to prevent it from developing in the first place. But unfortunately, preventing disease is not the focus of most medical professionals, medical institutions, or pharmaceutical companies. Medical professionals are trained to treat disease, not prevent it. There's little incentive for them to try to prevent disease. And there's certainly not enough money in disease prevention to attract the attention of pharmaceutical companies. And since most research is funded by the pharmaceutical companies, when compared with drug research, relatively little research is being done on disease prevention. Consequently, many diseases are the result of iatrogenic treatments — treatments for other issues using drugs that injure the digestive tract as a side effect. Before we explore that in detail though, let's consider some other problems that need to be resolved.

One of the problems with modern medicine is that physicians are still being trained to consider every health problem as a separate issue.

This may be slowly changing, as we shall see in the next chapter, but currently it's a huge obstacle to the efficiency and effectiveness of medical treatment. Anything that affects one part of the body affects all the rest of the body to some degree. For example, any problem with the digestive system affects every organ in the body in some way. The migraines, arthritis symptoms, and nausea that affect many MC patients are not separate issues — they're caused by the primary disease. Physicians need to start thinking in terms of the whole body whenever patients describe their symptoms, because it's all associated in one way or another.

How many lab tests are based on so-called "normal" ranges that were originally developed using skewed data?

Using so-called "normal" ranges that are not actually normal compromises the value of such tests and surely results in a lot of misdiagnosed and mistreated cases. Few things tend to be more misleading than lab tests that are based on incorrect normal ranges. This is a serious (and persistent) problem within the health care system, but no one seems to be concerned enough to attempt to correct it.

We've already discussed how the so-called "normal" ranges for magnesium were skewed by the improper selection of subjects who were used to establish those values. Apparently, as many as 80 % of the subjects who were considered to have normal magnesium levels when normal ranges for magnesium were being developed, were actually magnesium deficient. That means that the resulting "normal" range that was developed is biased toward the deficient side. The true normal range should be higher.

The TSH test that is used to assess thyroid function is another example of a biased "normal range" because the data seem to have been based on a test population that was called "normal" when many of them actually had undiagnosed hypothyroidism. How many other medical tests are sometimes incorrectly interpreted because they are based on skewed data?

Celiac disease is incorrectly described.

For some reason, the medical community continues to have a tough time understanding celiac disease. Though a description that appears to refer to the disease can be found in the medical literature written roughly 2,000 years ago, very little was learned about the disease until a Spanish physician published a book in 1922 in which he described the details of a pediatric case. Another doctor also described a case where eating bread or biscuits caused a child to have diarrhea. These observations inspired a Dutch physician to suspect wheat and he began doing experiments using a wheat-free diet. He published his first results in 1941, and at the International Congress of Pediatrics in New York City in 1947 he reported that bread or cookies made with wheat flour aggravate celiac disease. But because of bias, selective attention deficit disorder, or maybe due to the phase of the moon, the medical world refused to take his research discovery seriously.

So he solicited the help of a few colleagues who were able to develop a fecal fat test. By using that test they proved that removing wheat from the diet reduced the amount of unabsorbed fat in the stool. Furthermore they proved that reintroducing wheat into the diet of susceptible patients increased the fecal fat content in their stool. This information was brought to the attention of the International Congress of the International Pediatric Association in 1950.

But not surprisingly, publication of the results was delayed because the article was rejected by a prestigious American medical journal. Why is this not surprising? Because the medical authorities who are in a position to control the acceptance for publication of such articles (by peer-review) are generally resistant to any claim that contradicts current policy, regardless of how convincing the proof might be. And they tend to enforce this unwritten policy of status quo by disallowing the publication of such articles in prestigious, peer-reviewed journals. The article was finally published several years later in a Scandinavian medical journal.

Roughly a half-century later an American gastroenterologist and researcher had a similar experience when he tried to publish his research describing a testing method based on the detection of IgA antibodies to food sensitivities in stool samples. The medical community has traditionally used blood tests for screening for celiac disease. But the antibodies are produced in the intestines, not the blood, so the blood tests have very poor sensitivity in general. The stool test method is capable of detecting gluten sensitivity even before significant damage to the villi of the small intestine can be detected, and the procedure was granted a patent. But roughly twenty years later, the mainstream medical community still will not publish his medical proof, nor accept and endorse his tests, even though thousands of satisfied users have praised the accuracy and usefulness of the test results. If the stool tests were widely used by clinicians, the results could cut years off the diagnostic lag that typically occurs between the initial onset of clinical symptoms of gluten sensitivity and the point at which the damage to the villi is severe enough to qualify for an official diagnosis of celiac disease using current diagnostic methods.

But instead, the medical community continues to use primitive and obsolete diagnostic methods, so gluten-sensitive patients continue to suffer needlessly. They cannot receive an official diagnosis until the villa of their small intestine are almost totally flattened and destroyed. Furthermore, this unpublished research reveals that the inflammation that perpetuates microscopic colitis is due to food sensitivities (again, marked by antibodies in stool), and it has been demonstrated that removing those foods from the diet can control the symptoms. But mainstream medicine continues to treat these patients using obsolete methods.

The medical community must find and adopt an updated, accurate, and reliable way to diagnose celiac disease.

The diagnostic criteria currently used to diagnose celiac disease are far too limiting and because of the poor sensitivity of the tests that are used, an unacceptably high percentage of celiac disease cases are never diagnosed. No officially approved diagnostic test for non-celiac gluten sensitivity is even available, so that effectively prevents the "official" diagnosis of non-celiac gluten sensitivity. Even the most obvious symptoms of gluten sensitivity are sometimes overlooked, and more subtle symptoms are far less likely to be associated with gluten sensitivity. It's high time that clinicians are trained to recognize the symptoms of gluten sensitivity that they have been overlooking for many decades simply because they have inadequate training and no officially approved updated guidelines to follow.

Traditionally, physicians only consider gluten sensitivity as a possible diagnostic option when gastrointestinal symptoms such as diarrhea and bloating are present. But the first symptoms (and in some cases the only symptoms) of gluten sensitivity in many cases are neuromuscular disorders, including peripheral neuropathy (nerve damage that affects movement, sensation, or balance) and muscle inflammation (Hadjivassiliou et al., 1997, Hadjivassiliou, Grünewald, & Davies-Jones, 2002). If physicians were trained to recognize these symptoms, in many cases they could diagnose gluten sensitivity years earlier, thus preventing a lot of additional intestinal damage and patient suffering.

Microscopic colitis treatment is confounded by similar obsolete practices.

Mainstream medicine hasn't yet come to grips with all of the implications of celiac disease, so they're certainly not ready to take on a similar issue with microscopic colitis. After all, collagenous colitis was first described only about 40 years ago, so compared with celiac disease, microscopic colitis is still way back in the queue. And according to some authorities, even today, as many as approximately 19 out of 20 cases of celiac disease are never diagnosed because of the primitive and unrealistic diagnostic criteria that continue to be used by the medical community. Because MC can only be diagnosed by examining biopsy samples taken from the colon under a microscope, the disease faces even greater diagnostic challenges than celiac disease.

But there's also another issue here. It's now well accepted that changing the diet to avoid gluten is a complete (and preferred) treatment for celiac disease, with no need for any additional (medical) intervention. Celiac disease was the first inflammatory bowel disease ever medically described. It seems rather obvious that if a type of inflammatory bowel disease (celiac disease) can be completely controlled by diet changes then it's very likely that diet changes might also be effective for treating the other types of IBD. Perhaps the more complex types of IBD might require more complex diet changes than celiac disease, but diet changes should still be the proper primary approach for inflammation control.

So one would think that the medical community would be focusing it's research on investigating ways to control the other IBDs by methods that specifically (among other possible options) exclude gluten from the diet. At the very least they should be diligently trying to systematically rule out the option of using diet to treat the other IBDs. But instead they choose to focus on drug-based treatments. No one is interested in treating anything with diet changes, because there's no money in it for anyone in the industry, especially for the drug companies, where most research funding originates.

Mainstream medicine needs to change its focus on the use of drugs as the first line of treatment.

Allopathic medicine is clearly handicapped by a strong bias to use drugs to treat disease even when diet changes would be a better (much safer and more effective) approach. For evidence, one need look no further than the fact that while in medical school, physicians do not even receive enough training about diet-related health issues to be able to make intelligent decisions about their own health, let alone the health of patients who may have all sorts of dietary issues. While they are informed about ways in which issues such as hypertension, heart disease and diabetes, for example, can be affected by diet, the effects of diet on arguably the most important system of organs in the body, the digestive system, are rarely considered. Yet when the digestive system malfunctions, every organ in the body tends to suffer.

Gluten sensitivity can adversely affect the entire digestive tract.

Currently, celiac disease is medically described as a disease of the small intestine, when in fact, most celiacs also experience inflammation of the colon when exposed to gluten (Koskela, 2011). The disease was initially described over two thousand years ago, yet the definition has never been updated to recognize that the large bowel is also affected by the pattern of inflammation caused by exposure to gluten. The fact that the lining of the colon does not contain any villi does not necessarily diminish the degree of inflammation, but it prevents using biopsy samples taken from the colon to diagnose celiac disease, because by medical definition, celiac disease is not diagnosed by the degree of inflammation, but by the degree of villus flattening, thus arbitrarily ruling out using biopsy samples taken from the colon to diagnose celiac disease. And since the definition of celiac disease requires complete villus flattening (not partial flattening, and not the presence of inflammation just short of any villus flattening), many, many, patients who are sensitive to gluten remain without a diagnosis because they don't qualify for the diagnostic requirements, even though they are very sick. The medical community has failed them.

Likewise, microscopic colitis is usually associated with inflammation in both the small and large bowels, similar to celiac disease (Koskela, 2011). And because of the failure to include this information in the medical description of the disease, even many medical professionals incorrectly believe that MC is only associated with inflammation of the colon and does not affect the small intestine. Furthermore, experience shows that similar to Crohn's disease, virtually any organ in the digestive tract of a microscopic colitis patient can become inflamed because of the disease, but that's not included in the official definition of the disease, so most medical professionals are not aware of it. Is it any wonder then that the average physician typically has considerable difficulty understanding and treating the disease?

Are doctors shackled by their own modus operandi?

Physicians are stuck between a rock and a hard place because of the way that mainstream medicine has evolved over the last century. Mainstream medicine has evolved to allow only treatments based on published (peer reviewed) proof of concept. And ambulance-chasing lawyers have evolved to take advantage of the opportunity offered by that rigid style of treating patients by financially punishing any physicians who fail to follow that strict formula. Obviously this pretty much stifles creativity and any hope of using treatments other than the same old treatments that have performed so poorly in the past. Innovation is stifled. Just because an optional treatment works well doesn't mean that MDs can safely use it. Because of this, many physicians are unwilling to take chances on unproven treatments, because of the financial and professional risk. A method has to be published in a prestigious medical journal first, or they're afraid to try it, no matter how promising it might appear.

Most doctors don't understand food sensitivities.

And most physicians don't understand the sometimes subtle differences between food allergies, food sensitivities, and other gastrointestinal issues well enough to be able to distinguish one from the others. This isn't just my opinion — it's backed up by a study sponsored by several regulatory agencies of the U. S. government, including the Food and Drug Administration, Food and Nutrition Service of the U.S. Department of Agriculture, and National Institute of Allergy and Infectious Diseases.[230] The study clearly demonstrated the general lack of un-

207

derstanding by medical professionals. The study was also sponsored by organizations not affiliated with the government, including the Asthma and Allergy Foundation of America, Egg Nutrition Center, Food Allergy Research & Education, International Life Sciences Institute North America, International Tree Nut Council Nutrition Research & Education Foundation, National Dairy Council, National Peanut Board, and the Seafood Industry Research Fund.

The study concluded that because the medical community does not have adequate testing methods available (nor presumably, adequate training), the symptoms of food allergies are typically misinterpreted. Furthermore, because of these shortcomings, the actual prevalence of food allergies is unknown. So it's no wonder that food sensitivities are typically not even on the radar of most clinicians when diagnosing patients who complain of digestive system symptoms. This is a problem that is unlikely to be corrected before the medical schools begin to include proper dietary and food allergy training and food allergy and intolerance testing and treatment in their curriculum.

The concept of autoimmune reactions tends to be ambiguous, confusing, and generally misunderstood.

The term "autoimmune" is generally confusing because the medical community tends to give the impression that autoimmune diseases are due to reactions not only against tissues in the body, but triggered either by some mysterious unknown antigen or by certain cells of the body itself. That's simply not true.

Autoimmune reactions are always due to an outside antigen and when exposure to that antigen is removed, the autoimmune reaction will stop. The cause of the reaction is sometimes gluten or some other food sensitivity, or it may be due to a drug or something else, but it is virtually never due to cells that are part of the body itself.

The medical community is doing patients a grave injustice by hiding the fact that so-called autoimmune reactions can be easily stopped in many cases simply by avoiding the exogenous antigen that is triggering the reaction. In some cases, tracking down the cause of the reaction may not be easy, but in most cases it will turn out to be gluten or some other food sensitivity.

Except in Emergencies, antibiotics should not be given to children younger than two years of age.

Researchers studied antibiotic use in a group of children who were obese at four years of age (Scott et al., 2016).[231] They concluded that children younger that two years of age who received three or more antibiotic treatments had an increased risk of early childhood obesity. The risk increased as the number of antibiotic treatments increased.

The beef industry has been well aware of this fact for many years. For decades they have used antibiotics to help fatten cattle. Antibiotics have also been used to help fatten chickens for many years. Yet until relatively recently, doctors seemed stymied by the trend toward increasing childhood obesity, as they handed out more and more antibiotic prescriptions, sometimes for trivial ailments. So what does this suggest for the rest of us, who are older than two years of age? The implications are not good.

The concept of small intestinal bacterial overgrowth (SIBO) is exploited by many naturopaths and alternative practitioners.

This is strictly my opinion, but I've maintained all along that the gut biome of any individual is determined by diet, environment, and digestive efficiency. Whether or not any of the bacteria in our gut produce hydrogen, or methane, or whatever, is determined by our diet, our surroundings, and the efficiency of our digestion (unless we interrupt the process with an antibiotic).

Antibiotics will, of course, disrupt the numbers and the balance among gut bacteria, but over the course of a few weeks or months, the intestinal biome will tend to slowly return to basically it's original condition, again depending on diet, environment, and digestive efficiency. SIBO does exist, but it's a self-correcting condition that's exploited by many medical professionals who see it as an opportunity to make a lot of money by taking advantage of people's fears.

Yes, it's possible to have an intestinal infection that may need to be treated, but that's another matter entirely. Virtually everyone has SIBO when their MC is active, and it resolves when their MC is controlled, without any additional intervention, as digestion efficiency improves. Treating "SIBO" virtually never provides any long-term benefits for MC patients. Any perceived benefits will fade within a few days as the gut biome returns to homeostasis (a state of stability determined by prevailing conditions). But treating SIBO provides a very profitable source of income for many practitioners, even though it's usually a waste of time and money for the patient.

Acid reflux and GERD seem to be on the increase.

Reflux is almost always caused either by certain foods in the diet, or by medications. The use of certain medications is often overlooked as a cause of esophageal irritation. Published case studies show that over 100 drugs have been shown to cause esophageal injury and many of them are very often prescribed for various purposes. Many are non-prescription supplements or medications. These drugs include (but are not limited to) aspirin/NSAIDs, doxycycline, bisphosphonates, ascorbic acid/vitamin C, chemotheraphy agents, ferrous sulfate, nitroglycerine, anticholenergics, benzodiazepines, and many others (Tutuian, 2010).[232]

Some of these drugs promote reflux or GERD by decreasing the lower esophageal sphincter's clinching strength. We've already discussed how PPIs tend to do that, so of course they must be added to the list. It's ironic that they're often specifically prescribed to treat or prevent esophageal injury, when in fact, they can cause that very problem. And some drugs cause esophageal problems by affecting motility and or perception when swallowing.

The bisphosphonates carry additional serious risks.

Similar to proton pump inhibitors, they cause the very problem that they are prescribed to treat. The bisphosphonates increase bone density by preventing the body from resorbing old dead bone cells.[233] This deceives the tests that are used to measure bone density, because old dead bone is harder than normal, living bone. So based on test results, both the patient and the doctor mistakenly believe that the drug is helping to make stronger bones.

But the sad truth is just the opposite. The most dangerous effect of the bisphosphonates is the fact that new bone cells cannot be formed unless dead bone cells are removed first. So after a few years, the bones of bisphosphonate users become more and more brittle as dead bone tissue accumulates, while the formation of new bone cells continues to be blocked.

This is the reason why taking bisphosphonates is now limited to approximately a 5-year period — if patients use the drugs for a period of time much longer then 5 years, so many of them begin to have hip fractures that the drug companies become sitting ducks for lawsuits. By labeling the use of the drugs for a limit of 5 years, they hope that this will keep the cost of lawsuit payouts down to a level where the drug is still profitable for them.

The bisphosphonates are definitely not designed to benefit patients — they're designed to inflate drug company profits, while totally disregarding major problems with the drugs. And the doctors prescribing them either don't understand the risks, or they choose to look the other way, and hope that everything will somehow turn out OK.

Too many common drugs damage the mucosal lining of the gastrointestinal tract.

Some of these lesions can be difficult to distinguish from the damage caused by gastrointestinal disease. Yet the use of these drugs continues while everyone tries to ignore the risks. Surgical pathologists are well aware of the damage often done to the lining of the GI tract by commonly-prescribed drugs (De Petris et al., 2014).[234] One has to wonder why the routine use of these drugs continues. We've already discussed some of the drugs that are known to damage the esophagus. Now let's consider other parts of the GI tract that may be damaged by drugs.

According to Parfitt and Driman, (2007) even low doses of NSAIDs may cause ulcers, necrosis, or erosion of the mucosal lining of the stomach in up to 20 % of regular users.[235] And yet NSAIDs remain one of the most commonly-used groups of medications. Pathologists refer to the type of stomach injury caused by NSAIDs as reactive gastropathy, and this is a very common finding/diagnosis for biopsies of the stomach. According to Wallace, (1997) even though various approaches have been tried to reduce the degree of damage caused by NSAIDs to the gastrointestinal system, few methods have been successful in significantly reducing the risk of damage.[236]

PPIs are iatrogenic drugs.

The number of drug safety risks and warnings by the FDA that these drugs have collected over the years makes one wonder why they haven't been removed from the market.[237] They certainly should be. It has been known for years that they put the user at increased risk for the development of an intestinal bacterial infection (C. diff especially), chronic magnesium deficiency, osteoporosis, and fractures of various types. They interfere with the use of certain blood thinners (clopidogrel).[238] And more recently they have been shown to cause kidney disease (Lazarus, Chen & Wilson, 2016).[239]

Many, many patients have developed serious health issues that they didn't expect, after using these drugs for a while. After they have been used for more than a couple of weeks, weaning off PPIs typically becomes very difficult because of the well-known acid rebound effect they cause which usually makes the symptoms for which the drug was prescribed worse than they were before the drug was used (Reimer, Søndergaard, Hilsted & Bytzer, 2009).

Yet doctors continue to prescribe this class of drugs, disregarding the risks. According to the FDA, the label on over-the-counter PPIs recommends using the drug for only 14 days, and says that the treatment regimen should be used no more than three times per year. And yet according to statistics, the much stronger prescription version is typically used by the average patient for 6 months. And many patients use PPIs for a much longer period. Many MC patients feel that their MC was initially caused by a PPI, and published research backs them up (Masclee, Coloma, Kuipers & Sturkenboom, 2015, Law, Badowski, Hung, Weems, Sanchez & Lee, 2017).[240, 241]

Dr. Malcolm Kendrick, a Scottish physician, writes a blog in which he points out that PPIs double the risk of dying from heart disease (Kendrick, 2016, September 21).[242] This observation is supported by published research (Shah et al., 2015).[243] The research paper even specifically points out that use of the blood thinner clopidogrel does not diminish the risk increase from PPI use. Furthermore, the researchers point out that when H2 blockers are used instead of PPIs, a similar increase in the risk of dying from a heart attack does not occur. Dr Kendrick notes that PPIs suppress nitric oxide production, and the less nitric oxide you have in circulation, the more likely you are to die from cardiovascular disease. The process by which PPIs suppress nitric oxide is chemically rather complex, but it is explained in scientific language in a research paper by Cooke and Ghebremariam, (2011).[244] Evidently, a big part of the reason why PPIs increase the risk of heart attack is due to the magnesium-depleting characteristic of PPIs.

In addition to these problems, PPIs are generally thought to cause fundic gland polyps (the fundus is the upper part of the stomach). Research shows that 17 % to 35 % of PPI users develop these polyps after 12 months of use (Freeman, 2008).[245] Pediatric users of PPIs have been found to develop polyps after only 6 months of use(Freeman, 2008).

Normally, if a patient's stomach contains a Helicobacter pylori colony, the bacteria tend to populate only the lower part of the stomach (the antrum). But long-term use of PPIs tends to aggravate the bacteria, causing them to also populate the upper part of the stomach (the fundus), leading to an increase in gastritis. Since that's a known risk factor for stomach cancer, some authorities are concerned that long term PPI use might promote the development of stomach cancer.[246]

And in chapter 9, we will see how recent research has proven that PPIs more than double the risk of developing stomach cancer. Surely in view of all this evidence, there's no doubt by now that PPIs are clearly a class of iatrogenic drugs that should be removed from the market. Notably, the increased cancer risk associated with PPIs is not associated with H2 blockers, so they can be safely used for treating GERD symptoms.

Olmesartan (Benicar) is an angiotensin II receptor inhibitor used to treat high blood pressure.

According to De Petris et al. (2014) Benicar can cause collagenous gastritis, lymphocytic gastritis, or collagenous enteritis (either individually or combined), which may be indistinguishable (under a microscope) from the effects of celiac disease. Because the cellular changes due to microscopic colitis are so similar to the cellular changes caused by celiac disease, presumably this implies that Benicar can also cause cellular changes in the stomach and small intestine that are similar to the damage caused by MC. This suggests that the use of Benicar may lead to MC. In a small study done at the Mayo Clinic, Rubio-Tapia et al., (2012) concluded, "Olmesartan may be associated with a severe form of sprue-elike enteropathy. Clinical response and histologic recovery are expected after suspension of the drug" (p. 732).[247]

Many people believe (or maybe they hope) that by taking enteric coated aspirin (or other NSAIDs) they can avoid the gastrointestinal damage often caused by NSAIDs.

But De Petris et al. (2014) points out that enteric coatings simply transfer the damage to farther down the gastrointestinal tract. They note that enteric coatings may spare the stomach, but NSAIDs still cause ulcers and erosion damage throughout the small intestine. And the damage is especially common at the two ends of the small intestine, the beginning of the duodenum and the terminal ileum. According to an older article in The New England Journal of Medicine, 47 % of the patients in a study of rheumatoid arthritis patients who were taking NSAIDs, had small intestinal ulcers (Allison, Howatson, Torrance, Lee, & Russell, 1992).[248]

Certain drugs are known to damage the small intestine.

These drugs, including NSAIDs, Azathioprin Imuran), Olmesartan (Benicar), Colchicine (Colcrys), Ipilimumab (Yervoy), and Mycophenolate (CellCept) are known to cause small intestinal villus atrophy (De Petris et al., 2014). Of course villus atrophy is the cause of malabsorption problems and is a well-known diagnostic criterion of celiac disease, so this type of intestinal damage is very detrimental for one's overall health.

Some cleanout solutions used as a prep for a colonoscopy exam can damage the colon.

Sodium phosphate is known to cause ulcers (De Petris et al., 2014). Yet it is used as a cleanout solution to prepare for a colonoscopy and as an additive to many foods. Gluteraldehyde and hydrogen peroxide can cause colitis (De Petris et al., 2014). Gluteraldehyde is used as a disinfectant for cleaning endoscopes. Improper cleaning can result in enough remaining in the endoscope to damage the colon during the next use. NSAIDs, for example, can either cause injury directly, or cause further aggravation of IBDs or diverticulitis. They are well known for adversely affecting MC.

All in all, the use of many of these drugs is so widespread that the possibility exists that drugs might be responsible for all cases of microscopic colitis. That would make MC exclusively an iatrogenic disease.

Summary.

Physicians are trained to treat disease, not prevent it. Most research is funded by the pharmaceutical companies, so it's biased toward drug treatments, rather than dietary treatments. The so-called normal ranges of some tests are apparently skewed , and need to be corrected.

About 2,000 years after it was first described, celiac disease is still poorly diagnosed and poorly understood by many physicians, so it's not surprising that microscopic colitis has similar issues. In general, medical professionals don't understand food sensitivities. That important subject needs to be included in their training in medical school.

The definition of autoimmune diseases needs to be revised. It's currently misleading and confusing, especially for patients.

Many drugs used to treat various conditions are known to damage the digestive system. Over 100 drugs are known to cause damage to the esophagus alone. So many drugs are known to damage the digestive system in ways that are difficult or impossible to distinguish from the damage caused by disease, that there is a possibility that most cases of MC are caused by drugs, making it an iatrogenic disease.

Chapter 9

Recent Research

Recently published research challenges previous attitudes about IBDs.

Here we are over four decades since collagenous colitis was first described and there are still no medications labeled for any type of medical treatment for microscopic colitis in any of it's forms. One has to wonder why. The pharmaceutical companies surely realize by now that the disease is much more widespread than first believed, so the market potential should be large. So either they don't consider the market worth pursuing, (that is, they have decided that the cost of getting FDA approval of a new label would be too expensive to justify by the likely increase in sales volume), or they have another reason (which is not immediately apparent). There are drugs labeled to treat almost any disease one can imagine, but none labeled for microscopic colitis.

As far as new medical treatments are concerned, Uceris has become available since the first volume of *Microscopic Colitis* was published. It was primarily created for treating ulcerative colitis, so it's designed to become active after reaching the colon, and it's claimed to be especially active in the distal colon (the lower end of the colon), where ulcerative colitis is most commonly found. So it's not ideally suited for treating MC, which is usually found to be more prominent in the right-side colon and the terminal ileum (the lower end of the small intestine). But patients using Uceris to treat MC symptoms report that Uceris seems to perform surprisingly well. And it has the added benefit of not being activated until the medication has passed entirely into the colon, so there is no systemic action that might affect other body organs. Which means that there is no need to taper the dose when ending a treatment (in order to prevent damage to the adrenals). But as is the case with other medications, it is not labeled to treat MC, so using it is strictly an off-label use.

What have researchers learned about microscopic colitis that they didn't know before?

One thing they have learned is that many patients have been right all along — microscopic colitis is incorrectly named, because it also affects the small intestine in over half of the cases (Bonagura et al., 2016).[249] In their research report, the researchers emphasize the importance of this "discovery", by proposing the name "lymphocytic enterocolitis". Their report concludes with the observation that MC often involves the entire gastrointestinal track, something that many MC patients have been aware of for decades.

> In conclusion, MC is frequently associated with mild duodenal damage. This association may suggest the existence of a "microscopic enterocolitis", and specifically of a "lymphocytic enterocolitis", that involves the entire gastrointestinal tract. It is advisable to perform a colonoscopy with biopsies in all patients with type I Marsh-Oberhuber duodenal damage and symptoms as chronic diarrhea, abdominal or epigastric pain, loss of weight, after exclusion of standard causes. (p. 310)

So gastroenterologists (those who bother to keep up with current research), are finally on the same page as knowledgeable patients, and they may be in a much better position to be able to begin to understand the disease. Some of the best news regarding the medical community's understanding of MC, and their treatment programs for inflammatory bowel disease can be seen in current trends at some of the medical education institutions. Medical educators are becoming aware of the growing trend among patients who have gastrointestinal symptoms to request dietary treatments from their gastroenterologists. Currently, gastroenterologists either have inadequate training in dietary treatment methods, or they have been forced to learn the details of diet-based treatments on their own. As a result, most GI specialists either tend to deny that diet changes can be helpful in the treatment of IBDs or they have their own personal views of which diet changes might be helpful, and there are no established dietary treatment guidelines supported by the gastroenterological organizations. This situation obviously leads to a lot of frustration and confusion among patients.

But a change of attitude seems to be on the way. For example, at the University of Michigan, multidisciplinary-based treatments are being developed that will involve the participation of specially-trained dietitians and behavioral therapists, in treatment programs coordinated with gastroenterologists for treating issues such as celiac disease.[250] The goal is to provide optimum care for patients by integrating the skills of multiple medical professions, while ensuring collaboration so that everyone involved is on the same page. This change is long overdue in light of the long-term trend in medicine toward more specialization (and seemingly less collaboration among the various specialists involved in the various treatments prescribed for each patient). Similar programs are being developed at other institutions.[251]

Over the years, the trend toward more specialization in medicine has created an atmosphere of unnecessary complexity and increasingly inefficient use of resources in the treatment of many medical conditions. And from the patient's viewpoint this type of relatively uncoordinated treatment environment causes too much confusion, wastes too much time, continues to add to the escalating costs of medical care, and far too frequently ends in less than satisfactory resolution of the patient's health issues. So these new developments in medical training methods are encouraging.

The brain fog that often develops with MC may have a sinister side.

MC appears to be associated with neurodegenerative diseases such as Alzheimer's, Parkinson's and amyotrophic lateral sclerosis, (ALS). This association hasn't yet been proven, but all of these diseases seem to have a gastrointestinal connection. For example, patients who have Parkinson's disease have been shown to have different gut biomes than people who do not have the disease. Furthermore, Parkinson's patients have been shown to have had gastrointestinal issues decades before their Parkinson's symptoms developed.

According to The Michael J Fox Foundation, almost 80 % of Parkinson's patients have constipation that usually begins several years prior to the development of Parkinson's symptoms (Dolhun, 2014, December 08).[252] Furthermore, not only do Parkinson's patients have altered gut biomes, but Parkinson's patients with different types of motor symptoms, have unique populations of gut bacteria that coordinate with the types of symptoms. For example, Parkinson's patients with more severe balance and gait problems have more Enterobacteria than others.

All Parkinson's patients have fewer Prevotella bacteria than normal people (Ghaisas, Maher, & Kanthasamy, 2016).[253] So do autistic children, incidentally. Interestingly, in normal people, this bacterium usually helps to produce thiamine and folate vitamins. Perhaps this is a clue.

The Michael J Fox Foundation also points out that a protein that's found in clumps in the brains of all Parkinson's disease patients (known as alpha-synuclein) can be found in certain other locations in the body outside of the brain, including the enteric nervous system —the nerves that control the digestive system, sometimes called the second brain (Dolhun, 2014, December 08). The question yet to be answered is whether alpha-synuclein might develop first in the gut and then eventually spread to the brain where it causes motor symptoms.

Recalling part of our discussion back in chapter 3, we know that Parkinson's patients have lower vitamin D levels than people who don't have Parkinson's, (Kwon et al., 2016). And we know that vitamin D deficiency may be a common cause of delayed gastric emptying in untreated Parkinson's patients (Kwon et al., 2016). And as discussed previously, we recognize that magnesium deficiency might also contribute to delayed stomach emptying.

Could these neurodegenerative diseases be consequences of decades of chronic vitamin D and magnesium deficiencies?

Looking at the associations of neurodegenerative diseases with decades of digestive disorders that are often connected with, and may be caused by vitamin D and magnesium deficiencies, suggests to me that these syndromes may not be diseases — they might be symptoms of ignoring chronic vitamin D and magnesium deficiencies for decades.

The brain fog that's often associated with MC certainly illustrates the ability of digestive system inflammation to cause serious neurological problems. And the fact that resolving MC symptoms resolves brain fog suggests that resolving these chronic deficiencies may be the key to preventing the development of neurodegenerative diseases.

If the deficiencies continue to remain untreated as the decades pass, then whether or not a neurodegenerative disease may develop is likely to be determined by the individual's predisposing genes. In other words, genetics will determine which type or types of neurodegenerative issues may develop due to unresolved nutrient deficiencies. At this point, this is strictly a theory. Time will tell whether or not it will eventually be proven by medical researchers to be valid.

In support of my theory, however, I would point out that magnesium has been shown to prevent the clumping of alpha-synuclein (Golts et al., 2002).[254] So a chronic magnesium deficiency would surely allow a buildup of clumps of alpha-synuclein.

Therefore a magnesium supplement such as magnesium threonate (which is capable of crossing the blood/brain border) might prove to be helpful for preventing the clumping of alpha-synuclein in the brain.

But again, this is unproven speculation at this point. To add to the support for this theory however, note that vitamin D and vitamin D receptors have been shown to be important in the treatment of Alzheimer's and Parkinson's disease (Butler et al., 2011).[255] Both Alzheimer's and Parkinson's patients are known to have lower vitamin D levels than the general population (Zhao, Sun, Ji, & Shen, 2013).[256]

There may also be a connection between IBDs and neurodegenerative diseases by way of MTHFR gene mutations (which cause methylation issues).

But this is a separate issue and a hugely complex subject that is poorly understood by most physicians, including gastroenterologists and most other medical specialists. But the fact that methylation issues are common with MC and other IBDs, and often complicate recovery, and they frequently result in neurodegenerative symptoms for IBD patients, certainly illustrates that there is a strong connection.

Zonulin has been found to affect non-celiac gluten sensitivity (NCGS) patients almost as much as as it affects celiacs.

Discovered less than two decades ago, zonulin is the protein in the blood that apparently is the primary means by which the body modulates the tight junctions in the epithelium of the intestines in order to regulate intestinal permeability (as discussed in chapter one on page 6). In order to verify the extent to which zonulin is affected by gluten in NCGS patients, a comparison study was conducted (Barbaro et al., 2015).[257] In the study, healthy controls showed an average zonulin level of 0.007 ng/mg (0.0175 nmol/l). It was found that celiacs averaged a zonulin level of 0.033 ng/mg (0.0825 mmol/l)). And in NCGS patients the average zonulin level was very similar at 0.030 ng/mg (0.075 mmol/l).

Interestingly, the researchers found that when a GF diet was followed, the average zonulin level decreased significantly for celiacs, or anyone who had at least one HLA-DQ2 gene, but it did not decrease significantly for NCGS patients, or anyone who did not have an HLA-DQ2 gene. What does this tell us? It suggests that most NCGS patients have additional food sensitivities besides gluten that must be avoided in order to prevent the production of antibodies. Not surprisingly, this simple observation seems to have escaped the mainstream medical community.

A new organ has been classified.

The membrane that holds the intestines and other abdominal organs in position (known as the mesentery) has long been ignored by physicians.

But it was recently classified as an official organ (MacDonald, 2017, January 3).[258] And researchers have made some surprising discoveries about it. Sideri et al. (2015) discovered that the fat cells in the mesentery are able to regulate inflammation in Crohn's disease and ulcerative colitis.[259] The discovery of a connection between mesentery fat and inflammation of the epithelium of the colon is rather surprising. What this discovery might lead to (if anything) remains to be seen.

Gut biomes may be changing continually.

If you read much of the information available on this topic (especially if you consider the sales pitches offered by the probiotics industry) you might conclude that there is a certain balance of gut bacteria that you should strive to achieve and maintain in order to promote good overall health.

But the truth is that an optimum gut biome is a very individual matter. Our gut biome is determined by the foods that we eat, how well we digest them, whether or not we have had any antibiotics lately, and our environment (that is, which species of bacteria are available in our food and our surroundings).

Research shows that gut biomes vary significantly, especially for IBD patients, and they are often in a state of change (Halfvarson et al., 2017).[260] In a study of 137 individuals, 49 of which had Crohn's disease, 60 had ulcerative colitis, 4 had LC, 15 had CC, and 9 were healthy controls, the researchers determined that patients who had ileal Chron's disease had gut biomes that varied the most from healthy controls.

Interestingly, the gut biomes of some of the patients who had colonic Crohn's disease or UC did not vary significantly from the biomes of healthy controls. But the biomes of LC and CC patients did vary significantly from those of healthy controls in the study. The researchers noted that there is a wide range in the gut bacteria balances for IBD patients, even when they are in remission (but again, remember that in my personal opinion, that range is determined mostly by their diet.

Groundbreaking research has been published that may change the way that gastroenterologists treat IBDs.

In a small study conducted at Seattle Children's Hospital and Children's Healthcare of Atlanta, researchers proved that they can resolve active Crohn's disease and ulcerative colitis among pediatric patients by diet alone.[261] The researchers were able to bring the subjects into remission by using the specific carbohydrate diet (SCD). So now proof has been published that diet can be used to attain remission of patients who have either of the three most well-known types of IBD, celiac disease, Crohn's disease, and ulcerative colitis. Can published proof that diet can be used to resolve the symptoms of MC be far behind?

Of course this was only a small study, so the results will have to be verified by larger studies. But in this study, which was only 12 weeks long, 8 of the 10 patients who finished the regimen achieved remission by dietary changes alone (Novel diet shows promise in treating children with Crohn's disease and ulcerative colitis. 2016, Dec 28).[262] So now, gastroenterologists can no longer claim that diet has no effect on IBDs. If you hear that from your doctor you know immediately that she or he is not keeping up to date with research. But remember, kids heal faster than older people. That 12-week trial wouldn't have worked as well with older patients. More time would surely have been required.

Actually, complementary and alternative treatments have long been widely used for treating pediatric IBD cases for years, in as many as 30 % to 70 % of cases.

When researchers sent surveys to pediatric IBD centers in Atlanta, Houston, and San Francisco inquiring about treatments between 2001 and 2003, they found that complementary and alternative medicine (CAM) treatments were used by approximately 50 % in the IBD group and 23 % in the chronic constipation group (Wong et al., 2009).[263] In the IBD group, about 25 % used spiritual interventions and about 25 % used nutritional supplements. The data indicated that 43.6 % of all IBD patients used both prescription medications and CAM treatments. There were also some patients in both the IBD and the chronic constipation groups who used CAM treatments only, with no prescribed medications or other intervention. Interestingly, the patients in the IBD group who used CAM therapy felt that the CAM therapy benefited their condition almost as much as the conventional medical treatments, which showed a perceived benefit rating that averaged approximately 80 %. So it's likely that CAM treatments will probably be more widely used in the future.

The safety and efficacy of long-term use of low-dose budesonide has been established.

Researchers in Sweden have published proof that using budesonide at 4.5 mg per day is safe and effective for treatment periods of at least a full year (Münch et al., 2016).[264] Normally, a budesonide treatment starting at 9 mg per day for a month and then continued for another month or so at progressively-reduced dosages provides remission for most patients. But over 80 % of patients relapse when that initial budesonide treatment is ended. Münch et al. (2016) demonstrated that a budesonide treatment does not have to be ended after just a few months. The researchers concluded that:

> *Budesonide at a mean dose of 4.5 mg/day maintained clinical remission for at least 1 year in the majority of patients with collagenous colitis and preserved health-related quality of life without safety concerns. Treatment extension with low-dose budesonide beyond 1 year may be beneficial given the high relapse rate after budesonide discontinuation.* (p.47)

But there is a downside to the use of corticosteroids — another reason not to use them to treat IBDs has been discovered.

Using corticosteroids may increase the risk of developing diabetes. By searching electronic health records of IBD patients, researchers have discovered that IBD patients who use glucocorticoid drugs for treatment are more than 3 times as likely to develop diabetes as those who do not use the drugs (Gastroenterology & Endoscopy News Staff, 2015, May 27).[265] They found that 20 % of the patients who used glucocorticoid drugs developed diabetes, while only 5.8 % of those who did not use the drugs developed diabetes.

Light may affect MC.

The inflammation that is claimed to cause MC is due to the infiltration of lymphocytes into the mucosa of the intestinal lining of the colon. These lymphocytes are known as T cells, and they may be either "killer" T cells or "helper" T cells. T cells are also very abundant in the skin because the epithelia of the skin is similar to the epithelia of the intestines, except that it does not have a mucosal layer. Phan, Jaruga, Pingle, Bandyopadhyay and Ahern (2016) have discovered that not only does the skin use ultraviolet light to produce vitamin D, but the UV light also increases the motility of T lymphocytes in the skin.[266] Low-level blue light triggers the production of hydrogen peroxide by the T cells, which is subsequently used to activate certain enzymes that also enhance motility.

But whether or not this discovery affects the lymphocytes in the intestines so that it might affect MC remains to be seen. Obviously, specific research regarding the disease is needed.

Probiotics continue to be a subject of research studies for digestive issues.

In the past, probiotics have been recommended by many gastroenterologists as part of a treatment regimen for MC, But in mid-December of 2016, the American Gastroenterological Association Institute decided to recommend against the use of probiotics for the medical management of microscopic colitis, reversing their previous position (Nguyen, Smalley, Vege, Carrasco-Labra, & the Clinical Guidelines Committee, 2016, December 18).[267] A few months prior to that, a Russian team of researchers published data with glowing conclusions about the success of a treatment program for IBS patients using a commercially-produced probiotic (Wild, 2016, March 21).[268]

The study, which involved treatment twice daily with either 250 mg of a probiotic available in Russia called Florasan-D (which is a combination of Bifidobacterium bifidum, Bifidobacterium longum, Bifidobacterium infantis and Lactobacillus rhamnosus), or a placebo, involved only 64 subjects and a treatment period of only 28 days. Roughly half the participants in the study were claimed to have diarrhea-predominant IBS and the other half were rated as having constipation-predominant IBS. Success at treating SIBO was measured by means of lactulose breath testing (which is a rather dubious way to measure the success of any treatment) and a questionnaire which rated clinical symptoms and stool consistency.

The results showed that on the average, for the subjects taking the probiotic product, abdominal pain decreased, flatulence decreased, the number of bowel movements decreased, and stool consistency improved from type 6 to 4 on the Bristol Stool Chart.

But wait — the subjects taking a placebo also showed similar improvements (though the report failed to emphasize that). And naturally, all of the subjects who showed signs of SIBO (based on a lactulose breath test) at the start of the treatment regimen, showed complete resolution (again, based on lactulose breath test results). All in all, the interpretation of the results seems to be somewhat arbitrary, and biased toward a perceived effectiveness of the probiotic, even though actual medical proof of efficacy was lacking.

In general, considering patient experiences, the accumulated experience of many MC patients indicates that treatments with probiotic products seldom provide any useful benefits for most patients. And in some cases, they cause major flares. For most patients, most probiotic products seem to make no difference, providing neither benefits nor detriments, which means that they are probably a waste of money in most cases.

Limit the use of medications with anticholinergic properties.

Research has shown that they are associated with dementia and Alzheimer's disease.[269] And the effects appear to be cumulative, so that simply avoiding their use from time to time will not prevent the long-term risks. The more they are used, the greater the increased risk of developing dementia and Alzheimer's disease. This class of drugs includes first-generation antihistamines, tricyclic antidepressants, commonly-used sleeping pills, and other types of medications. This is important because some of the medications taken to treat MC fall into this category.

You'll probably be hearing about Tailored Leukapheresis Immunotherapy soon (if you haven't heard about it already).

This process is claimed to be a treatment for not only all IBDs (including MC), but all immune mediated inflammatory diseases. In other words, this patented treatment is claimed to be capable of treating all so-called autoimmune diseases, and it's currently being developed for commercial (medical) use (Targeted Immuno Therapies AB and Ferring Pharmaceuticals sign a strategic collaboration agreement for the treatment of IBD, 2016, January 11).[270] Discovered at the Karolinska Institutet (in Sweden), the treatment is claimed to remove inflammatory cells from the blood as they are on their way to the the the site of inflammation (Tailored Leukapheresis Treatment, n.d.).[271] The treatment is said to remove chemokines from the blood before they can reach the body's chemokine receptors at the inflammation site, thus preempting activation of the receptors and thereby interrupting the inflammation process. During the treatment, the patient's blood is passed through the machine, where the inflammatory cells are removed, and the blood is then returned to the body.

The treatment sounds impressive, and it probably will work as described. There's just one problem — like all the other medical treatments for immune system disorders, it treats the symptoms, but it does not treat the cause of the inflammation. The inflammation will begin to be regenerated as soon as the patient eats her or his first meal after the treatment. How much time will pass before this expensive and intrusive treatment will need to be repeated? . . . A week? . . . Two weeks? . . . Four weeks? Similar to dialysis treatments, the patient will be a regular customer for the rest of her or his life — not a very appealing arrangement for the patient, but very lucrative for the medical system.

Research into possible stem cell therapy to provide a permanent cure option for IBD is being studied.

But besides the ethical issues that must be considered, any type of stem cell therapy that might be successful would need to coordinate the transplantation of several different types of cells into intestinal tissue in order to accomplish the task. Currently, it's unlikely that researchers will be able to meet this challenge without a better understanding of the biotechnology involved. Nevertheless, the fact that researchers are publishing articles on this topic indicates that they are certainly investigating the possibilities (Hawkey et al., 2000, Flores et al., 2015).[272], [273] If any successful treatments are discovered, based on this technology, they will likely be developed in the distant future.

Soy contains peptides that act as natural bacteriocides.

While that's not surprising, some of the claims made by some of the researchers who have investigated this discovery are more than a little hard to believe, as they have not been verified by others (Dhayakaran, Neethirajan, & Weng, 2016).[274] For example, claims made by one of the researchers in an interview, such as "The compounds in soybeans, however, do not kill off all bacteria, just the bad ones, Neethirajan said", sound like unsubstantiated hype (Bueckert, 2016, April 26).[275] Furthermore, claims that these peptides will not be a problem for people who have a sensitivity to soy are strictly unproven speculation. When something sounds too good to be true, it usually is (too good to be true). That said, some of these soy isolates will probably be used as food additives in the future, adding to the risk of adverse reactions for people who are sensitive to soy and it's derivatives.

Fructose alters brain genes. (which can cause metabolism issues and inflammation).

This has been demonstrated by Meng et al. (2016) .[276] The researchers also discovered that a fatty acid, docosahexaenoic acid (DHA), is capable of undoing the brain damage caused by fructose. They did this by first training rats to escape from a maze, and then dividing them into three groups. The first group was given enough fructose (in their water) to be approximately equal to the amount a human would ingest if they drank about a liter of soda each day. The second group consumed the same amount of fructose plus DHA. The third group drank only plain water (no fructose or DHA).

After six weeks on the diet, when the rats ran the maze, the group that had received only the fructose took about twice as long to escape from the maze as the control group (those that drank only water). But the group that received fructose plus DHA had similar times to the control group, indicating that the negative effects of the fructose on the rats' memory had been effectively erased from their brains.

Interestingly, the rats on a high-fructose diet had significantly higher blood glucose, triglycerides, and insulin levels than the rats in the other two groups. In humans, this is often associated with obesity, diabetes, and other diseases. Meng et al. (2016) discovered that over 700 genes in the rats' brains that were associated with metabolism had been altered by the fructose. Additionally, they found that over 200 genes associated with cognizance and memory had been altered by the fructose. These genes also regulate inflammation (Wolpert, 2016, April 21).[277]

Thus it appears that the brain fog so often associated with MC may be due to the effects of fructose in the diet or a DHA deficiency, or both. DHA has been demonstrated to help IBD patients (Tabbaa, Golubic, Roizen, & Bernstein, 2013).[278]

We know that fructose is metabolized differently than sucrose in the human digestive system.

Rather than being digested by the digestive system similar to sucrose and other sugars, fructose has to be metabolized in the liver. Because of that difference, little to none of it can be burned as energy, so it is mostly stored as fat.

Fructose has been shown to increase the risk of pancreatic cancer because of the fact that many strains of pancreatic cancer use fructose to reproduce (Liu et al, 2010).[279] Fructose has also been shown to cause insulin resistance and to reduce pancreatic production of insulin (thus leading to the condition known as prediabetes) (Elliott, Keim, Stern, Teff, & Havel, 2002).[280] Additional recent research confirms this connection.

Drinking just one can of sugar-sweetened soda daily has been shown to increase the odds of developing the condition known as prediabetes.

An article published in 2016 by Ma et al. verified this.[281] In fact, one of the researchers involved in the study pointed out that someone who drinks a can of sweetened soda daily has about a 46 % increase in the risk of developing prediabetes (Thompson, 2016, November 10).[282]

For some unknown reason, the study did not consider the type of sugar involved (which makes their findings much less valuable), but it's common knowledge that fructose makes up a majority of the sugar in sodas (in the form of corn syrup and high-fructose-corn syrup). Apparently the researchers considered all common types of sugar to be equal, even though they are not.

A simple urine test has been developed to detect the ingestion of gluten.

With this test, based on the detection of gluten immunogenic peptides (GIP) in urine., as little as 50 mg of gluten in a meal can be detected as soon as four to six hours after eating, and the test can detect gluten ingestion up to two days later. In a study involving 58 celiac patients and 76 healthy controls, Moreno et al., (2017) demonstrated that the test was accurate and reliable.[283] They also found that about 50 % of the people who claimed to be following a gluten-free diet were actually still eating some gluten.

This test will probably have rather limited usefulness for MC patients however, since by four to six hours after ingesting any gluten they will probably already be reacting with typical MC symptoms, so they won't need to be told that they slipped up on their diet. The test might be useful in cases where an individual is unsure about the safety of their diet.

There has been a significant amount of research in recent years about how DNA methylation is associated with IBDS.

Some researchers feel that this technology may lead to better treatments and ways to select treatments that are specifically tailored for individual patients. The association of DNA methylation with IBD has been well established and is reasonably well understood (Karatzas, Gazouli, Safioleas, & Mantzarisa, 2014).[284] DNA methylation is an example of gene regulation by epigenetics. But despite exciting theories about the future of this technology, there is much work to be done before researchers will have enough data to support any productive results. Until then, much of the published information may sound promising, but a lot of it appears to be little more than smoke and mirrors added to a rehash of previously published research.

PPIs more than double the risk of developing stomach cancer.

To add to the long list of problems with PPIs, now Cheung et al. (2017) have shown that long-term use of PPIs significantly increases the risk of developing stomach cancer.[285] This is especially bad news because stomach cancer is currently the third leading cause of cancer deaths in the world. The cancer risk is actually associated with Helicobacter pylori bacteria. While about two-thirds of the world's population seem to be colonized by H. pylori bacteria, normally this doesn't result in any problems. In a small percentage of cases however, this can lead to the development of stomach cancer. Cheung et al (2017) found that even when the H. pylori bacteria were eradicated, the risk of stomach cancer (eventually) more than doubled (due to PPI use). This was a study of 63,397 patients, and the researchers also noted that the longer a patient used PPIs, the greater their risk of developing stomach cancer.

GERD appears to be an autoimmune-associated disease.

The damage caused by GERD to the esophagus is actually caused by cytokines, not gastric acid, as originally thought. This discovery was initially made back in 2009 when Souza et al were experimenting with rats, and this was mentioned on page 180 of the first edition of *Microscopic Colitis*.[286] In2016, Dunbar, Agoston, & Odze verified that cytokines also mediate the inflammation associated with GERD in humans.[287] Examination under a microscope of esophageal epithelial biopsy samples from GERD patients reveals the characteristic T Lymphocyte infiltration associated with MC and all other autoimmune-type syndromes. Though the researchers didn't recognize the implication, this suggests that food sensitivities and/or drug sensitivities may be the root cause of the inflammation associated with GERD.

Research verifies that the risk of developing an IBD is determined by certain gut bacteria and gene mutations.

Bacteroides fragilis, a human gut microbe, is known to produce immunomodulatory molecules that are capable of warding off the development of IBD. Chu et al. (2016) showed in a laboratory experiment that these molecules can protect mice from developing colitis when exposed to chemicals that normally cause colitis in other mice.[288] Normally (with normal ATG16L1 and NOD2 genes), this allows dendritic cells (DCs) to produce regulatory T cells that protect against colitis. But research by Chu et al. also showed that dendritic cells that are deficient in ATG16L1 genes did not produce regulatory T cells that protect against colitis. This suggests that gene mutations (polymorphisms of these genes) may be responsible for an increased risk of developing an IBD.

This was not mentioned in the research article, but from this evidence, we might also deduce that if Bacteroides fragilis are absent from the gut, then the risk of developing an IBD would be increased. That would imply that both gene mutations and altered gut microbiomes might be responsible for an increase in the risk of developing an IBD, either independently or in combination.

A recent study showed that up to 27 % of southern Europeans may be vitamin D Deficient.

Researchers estimate that up to one-third of the world's population is vitamin D deficient. And in some areas the problem is even worse. By combining the results of 107 individual studies done in Cyprus, Greece, France, Israel, Italy, Malta, Portugal, Spain, and Turkey, they found that a surprising number of individuals had very low Vitamin D levels (Manios et al., 2017).[289] The researchers discovered that :

20 % of infants had a vitamin D level below 10 ng/ml (25 nmol/l).

27 % of adolescents had a vitamin D level below 10 ng/ml (25 nmol/l).

16 % of adults had a vitamin D level below 10 ng/ml (25 nmol/l).

16 % of the elderly had a vitamin D level below 10 ng/ml (25 nmol/l).

The researchers noted that despite the sunny environment in southern Europe and the Mediterranean, vitamin D deficiency there is widespread. If Vitamin D deficiency is so prevalent in southern Europe, one naturally wonders how extensive the problem might be in Northern Europe and various other parts of the world.

Research with Helminths suggests that they may target mast cells as a means of inflammation suppression.

Vukman, Lalor, Aldridge, & O'Neill, (2016) were able to demonstrate that at least one type of helminth (Fasciola hepatica, also known as the common liver fluke or sheep liver fluke), secretes molecules that suppresses mast cell proliferation, thereby suppressing inflammation.[290] It has long been known that an infection with helminths would bring remission of Crohn's disease or ulcerative colitis symptoms, but conventional thinking was that the helminths brought relief from an IBD by simply distracting the immune system. According to the findings of this research, helminths are capable of actually suppressing inflammation by producing a substance that stops inflammation by preventing the proliferation of mast cells and by suppressing their degranulation.

This supports my theory (discussed on page 163–165 in chapter 5) that the inflammation associated with IBDs and other so-called autoimmune diseases may be primarily due to mast cells, and not lymphocytes, as claimed by the medical community. The lymphocytes may merely be innocent bystanders that are there in a supporting role.

In a laboratory setting, researchers have shown that certain food preservatives may promote obesity.

By utilizing stem cells, researchers discovered that some commonly-used chemicals can disrupt the production of certain hormones and their communication between the gut and the brain (Rajamani et al., 2017).[291] They were able to show that butylhydroxytoluene (BHT) which is an regularly added to cereals and other foods as a preservative, perfluoroctanoic acid (PFOA), which is a polymer used in certain types of cookware, and tributyltin (TBT), which is a compound commonly found in paint that seeps into water and is often found in seafood, acted as endocrine disruptors to interfere with communications between the gut and the brain. This could prevent the brain from receiving signals that it normally receives to help it decide when someone is full, so that they will stop eating. Since the research was done using stem cells, it's likely that this would apply mostly to unborn babies still in the womb. But it suggests an obesity problem that would be passed to future generations because of the endocrine disruption.

Titanium dioxide (Ti02) nanoparticles should be avoided by individuals who have an IBD.

Titanium dioxide nanoparticles are widely used as a white pigment in drugs and as a food additive. Ruiz et al. (2017) showed that people who have an IBD, or food sensitivities, or for some other reason have increased intestinal permeability (leaky gut), should avoid titanium dioxide nanoparticles.[292] The additive may make symptoms worse for such individuals.

Could fiber be protective of food allergies?

In an interesting experiment, Tan et al, (2016) showed that mice specially bred to be allergic to peanuts and then fed a high-fiber diet that was enriched with vitamin A, could tolerate peanuts.[293] They also found that they could transplant some of the gut bacteria from these mice into the intestines of mice that had a peanut allergy and were previously bacteria-free and they would also become able to tolerate peanuts, even though they were not fed a high-fiber diet. It will be interesting to see if this can be utilized to work in human subjects.

Polycomb-group proteins are being studied because of their epigenetic attributes.

The double helix arrangement that we know as DNA in the nucleus of each of our cells is organized and encased by special proteins known as histones. The resulting complex of protein and DNA is called chromatin.

Polycomb-group proteins are a family of proteins that are capable o modifying chromatin to enable epigenetic deactivation of certain genes. The cells in the intestinal epithelium are normally replaced by new cells about every four or five days. Regulating this process is a difficult job that's handled by polycomb. But Oittinen et al. (2017) have shown that this process (homeostasis) is dysregulated when either celiac disease or colorectal cancer are present, suggesting that the corruption of polycomb regulation of epithelial homeostasis may occur with any inflammatory disease.[294] Oittinen et al. (2017) have shown that when celiac disease or cancer is present, polycomb methylates histone proteins, which turns off certain genes epigenetically, resulting in a corruption of the normal homeostasis of the intestinal epithelium. That's a mouthful, but it may well hold the key to the basic cause of all IBDs.

Melatonin has been shown to be effective for treating GERD without any of the side effects of PPIs.

Melatonin is produced by the pineal gland (in the brain), and it helps to regulate sleep. It's also produced in enterochromaffin cells in the intestines, where it helps to regulate motility. Kandil, Mousa, El-Gendy, & Abbas, (2010) proved that melatonin can be used either alone or in combination with omeprazole to effectively treat GERD, without the side effects usually associated with the use of proton pump inhibitors.[295] They demonstrated that 3 mg of melatonin , taken once per day, was effective for treating GERD.

This discovery was taken a step further by de Oliveira Torres & de Souza Pereira, (2010) when they pointed out that most GERD patients have a sleep disorder due to a melatonin deficiency, and melatonin also controls the lower esophageal sphincter and acid secretion in the stomach.[296] The enterochromaffin cells in the intestines produce approximately 400 times as much melatonin as the pineal gland (in the brain). But the evidence shows that PPIs damage enterochromaffin cells. Therefore, it seems counterproductive to compromise the functioning of the primary source of melatonin. They concluded that melatonin is a far safer treatment for GERD, than PPIs.

Anti-TNF medications have been shown to be effective for treating MC.

While many gastroenterologists are reluctant to recommend treatments that are based on major diet changes to avoid inflammatory foods, they seem to have no qualms about prescribing powerful and risky drugs, such as the anti-TNF medications. By analyzing hospital records, Esteve et al. (2011) showed that anti-TNF medications are effective for treating MC cases that do not respond to conventional treatments.[297] This was supported by an article published by Park, Cave, & Marshall, in 2015.[298]

Do electromagnetic fields (EMF) affect MC?

Currently, there is a lot of speculation about how electromagnetic fields may be affecting various systems in the human body. We continue to add electronic devices into our nearby environment without knowing whether they might have some adverse effect upon our body. Many possibilities have been suspected, but so far, there has been no proof of any connection between EMF and any chronic diseases.

Nevertheless, suspicions of various effects continue. A synopsis of the prevailing thoughts on this issue can be found in a recently-published paper (Belyaev et al., 2016).[299]

The long-term effect of vitamin D level and disease symptoms of IBD patients has been documented.

During a 5-year research project, the vitamin D levels of 965 IBD patients were correlated with their symptoms and general disease status (Kabbani et al., 2016).[300] About 61.9 % of the group had Crohn's disease and the other 38.1 % had ulcerative colitis. Initially, 42 % of the patients had low vitamin D levels. Some took a Vitamin D supplement, so at the end of the study, only 28.5 % were found to have low vitamin D levels.

The researchers found that those patients who had the highest levels of vitamin D, needed less care and less medications in general, than those with the lowest levels. They noted that IBD patients with low vitamin D levels had worse disease activity, more pain, a higher need for medications, and a greater general need for the services of the health care system. The researchers concluded that "Low vitamin D levels are common in IBD patients and are associated with higher morbidity and disease severity, signifying the potential importance of vitamin D monitoring and treatment" (p. 712). And as discussed back in chapter 3, this is supported by other research.

Vitamin D helps to protect against the development of autoimmune diseases and cancer.

Antinuclear antibodies (ANA) are a particular type of antibody that attack naturally occurring proteins in the body. High ANA levels are associated with various types of autoimmune disease. Reexamining data from the National Health and Nutrition Examination Survey (NHANES), which was originally collected in 2001–2004, Meier, Sandler, Simonsick, and Parks (2016) determined that middle-aged and older people (in the U.S.) who had vitamin D levels that were deficient (below 10 ng/ml [25 nmol/l])were almost 3 times as likely (2.99 actually) to have an elevated ANA level as those who had a sufficient blood level of vitamin D (over 30 ng/ml [75 nmol/l]).[301]

Those with a vitamin D level between 10 ng/ml (23 nmol/l) and 30 ng/ml (75 nmol/l) were twice as likely to have an elevated ANA level (compared with those who had a sufficient vitamin D level). The researchers concluded that "Vitamin D deficiency in older adults may increase vulnerability to cancer by contributing to immune dysfunction." (Meier, Sandler, Simonsick, & Parks, 2016 . p. 1559).

Meeker, Seamons, Maggio-Price, & Paik (2016) have suggested that vitamin D should be used for protection against and treatment of IBD and colon cancer.[302] The researchers noted that the benefits of vitamin D in IBD and colon cancer have been verified by both human epidemiologic data and animal studies, and the majority of evidence supports the position that vitamin D has the potential to be an inexpensive and effective treatment for these issues.

Garland and Gorham, (2017) analyzed 15 earlier studies in 14 countries that involved the connection between colorectal cancer and vitamin D levels.[303] All but 2 of the studies showed that a higher vitamin D level was associated with a reduced likelihood of developing colorectal cancer. The conclusion reached by Garland and Gorham (2017) was that the correlation between higher vitamin D levels and reduced risk of colorectal cancer was strong. Those who had a blood 25(OH)D level of 30ng/ml (75nmol/l or better had at least a 33% reduced risk when compared with those who had a blood level of 5ng/ml (12.5 nmol/l).

Vitamin D deficiency is associated with all-cause mortality.

In a study involving 11,022 subjects, Schöttker et al. (2013) found that those who had a vitamin D blood level of less than 12 ng/ml (30 nmol/l) had a 71 %higher mortality risk when compare with those who had a vitamin D level greater than 20 ng/ml (50 nmol/l).[304] Those with a vitamin D level between 12 ng/ml (30 nmol/l) and 20 ng/ml (50 nmol/l) had a 17 % increased mortality risk when compared with those who had a vitamin D level greater than 20 ng/ml (50 nmol/l). Clearly, vitamin D levels below 12 ng/ml (30 nmol/l) should be avoided.

Vitamin D has been shown to help reduce clinical symptoms and the risk of relapse with ulcerative colitis.

Gubatan et al. (2017) has shown in a study that patients with vitamin D levels below 35 ng/ml (87.5 nmol/l) had a 46 % increased risk of having inflammation, and a 25 % increased risk of a relapse within 12 months.[305] In the study, the average vitamin D level of patients who relapsed was 29.5 ng/ml (73.8 nmol/l), while the average level of those patients who did not relapse was 50.3 ng/ml (125.8 nmol/l). Gubatan et al. (2017) concluded that "Serum levels of vitamin D of 35 ng/ml or less during periods of clinical remission increase the risk of UC relapse. Clinical trials to obtain vitamin D levels higher than this threshold should be considered."

The official guidelines from the *National Institutes of Health Office of Dietary Supplements* claim that 20 ng/ml (50 nmol/l) are "Generally considered adequate for bone and overall health in healthy individuals". They go on to claim that (in reference to levels higher than 50 ng/ml [125 nmol/l]) "Emerging evidence links potential adverse effects to such high levels, particularly >150 nmol/L (>60 ng/ml).

Really? One can't help but wonder exactly what adverse effects they are referring to. At any rate, these research data are strong evidence of the value of higher vitamin D levels than the official guidelines suggest, at least for IBD patients.

Vitamin D deficiency is associated with lower back pain.

In a study in India, Panwar, Valupadas, Veeramalla, and Vishwas, (in press) found that increasing severity of vitamin D deficiency was associated with a higher prevalence of lower back pain.[306] In other words, the lower the vitamin D level, the greater the likelihood that the patient would experience lower back pain.

Vitamin D has been associated with rheumatoid arthritis (RA).

In a study involving subjects in 15 countries, Hajjaj-Hassouni et al. (2017) found that patients whose vitamin D level was insufficient not only had more RA activity, but they also had more concurrent health issues, especially lung diseases and osteoporosis.[307] The researchers also noted that vitamin D levels were more likely to be insufficient when a corticosteroid was used, and when vitamin D was not supplemented.

Vitamin D supplementation may be helpful for all autoimmune diseases — it can decrease the seasonal relapse rate among multiple sclerosis patients, for example.

MS patients frequently suffer a relapse of symptoms in the late-winter/early spring period. Miclea et al. (2017) showed that annual relapse rates due to this seasonal effect can be reduced by about half by supplementing with vitamin D.[308] Supplementation of vitamin D is especially important during the late-fall/winter/early spring period when blood levels of vitamin D are normally at their lowest.

In a mouse-based study, researchers have identified a gene that is believed to protect the intestines from IBD.

They have also determined that a mutation to this gene corrupts the ability of the gene to provide protection against inflammation.

Normally, this gene (known as the Gatm gene) activates prompt replacement of the intestinal mucosal barrier against inflammation caused by bacteria, according to the study by Turer et al. (2017).[309] When that gene has been mutated, the ability to maintain mucosal integrity is compromised.

But the problem with this "discovery" is that the researchers make an initial assumption that IBDs are caused by the inability of the mucin glands in the crypts of our intestinal mucosa to produce mucin rapidly enough to prevent bacteria in the fecal stream from attacking the mucosa. When mucin mixes with water, it produces mucus, which normally lubricates and protects the surface of the intestinal mucosa.

While this is an interesting theory, researchers have theorized for decades that bacteria are the cause of IBD. But so far no one has been able to demonstrate that bacteria are indeed the cause of IBD, let alone prove that the reason why bacteria are the cause of IBD is because mucin production by the crypts in our mucosa is dramatically reduced. In fact, as any MC patient can attest, mucus production increases dramatically with most MC flares. It's a visible and very common symptom of active MC.

Despite all the elegant claims, this project is confounded at the outset by an inappropriate assumption. So it's speculation, not scientific fact. Contrary to the basis of that assumption, most MC patients seem to be quite capable of producing copious amounts of mucus.

Sometimes research articles can have stated conclusions that can be very misleading.

It seems that researchers are sometimes prone to interpreting the data somewhat arbitrarily. The conclusions reached in the resulting articles (published in various medical journals and other venues), sometimes seem to reflect a capricious convenience of the moment. Consider a project where researchers set out to determine whether or not vitamin D and calcium supplementation might reduce cancer risk.

This was a random-controlled trial (RCT), which is considered to be the gold standard for accuracy and reliability in medical research. This was a four -year RCT in which 2,302 healthy menopausal women who were 55 and older were given 2,000 IU per day of vitamin D and 1,500 mg per day of calcium. Their results were compared with a group of controls who received placebos. By the end of the trial, 106 women (43 who were receiving treatment and 63 who were receiving placebos) had developed at least one type of non-skin cancer.

But look at the conclusions of the publications that came out of this study. In 2016, Lappe, Travers-Gustafson, Garland, Heaney, Recker, & Watson presented a paper at the 2016 annual meeting of the American Public Health Association where they concluded that "Supplementing with 2000 IU/day of vitamin D3 and 1500 mg/day of calcium substantially reduced risk of all cancers combined".[310]

That sounds quite profound, until you also consider an article published about the same study in 2017 in the journal JAMA. The conclusion of this article appears to contradict the conclusion previously stated (Lappe et al., 2017).[311] A few additional researchers managed to get their names added to the article, but look at what they concluded in this article:

Conclusions and Relevance:

Among healthy postmenopausal older women with a mean baseline serum 25-hydroxyvitamin D level of 32.8 ng/mL, supplementation with vitamin D3 and calcium compared with placebo did not result in a significantly lower risk of all-type cancer at 4 years. Further research

249

> *is necessary to assess the possible role of vitamin D in cancer preven-*
> *tion.* (p. 1,234)

This is the same study and basically the same group of researchers, and yet the conclusions reached in the two articles are as different as night and day. Both articles are based on the same data, and yet the conclusions suggest a different outcome. They may well both be statistically accurate, but the way the conclusions are phrased appears to be very misleading. The first conclusion suggests that vitamin D and calcium supplementation is important for cancer prevention. The second conclusion implies that vitamin D and calcium supplementation is irrelevant for cancer prevention. That's not what it actually says of course, but the conclusion of the second article implies that vitamin D and calcium supplementation is irrelevant by stating that supplementation made no difference in the study (for subjects who were already vitamin D sufficient). It makes one wonder if these researchers were just playing games with statistics in order to get something published.

Furthermore, the project was not very well planned initially. It was blemished by the fact that 16 of the subjects in the treatment group and 10 in the placebo group developed kidney stones (referred to as "renal calculi" in the article). Additionally, 6 of the subjects being treated and 2 in the placebo group developed elevated serum calcium levels (hypercalcemia), a rather serious adverse event that can be life-threatening in some cases.

But these adverse events are not surprising, in light of the fact that the subjects in the treatment group were taking such a large calcium supplement every day, without taking extra magnesium to ensure that their magnesium levels were adequate to handle the relatively large calcium supplementation. In retrospect, the treatment group receiving relatively large calcium supplements should have been monitored to watch for insufficient magnesium levels and supplied with magnesium supplements to offset any excess calcium levels in the blood in cases where magnesium was needed.

But there is some very important insight to be discovered here. If you analyze the data from this research project, it becomes apparent that what the researchers actually proved was that while taking supplemental vitamin D is helpful for reducing the risk of cancer, taking a calcium supplement is not. Strangely, they failed to mention that simple but important point.

In a misguided research project designed to "prove" that taking supplemental magnesium provides no benefits against inflammation, researchers wasted their time and resources by beginning with an assumption that was either due to ignorance or intentional dishonesty.

The project got off to a great start when it was designed as a double-blinded, placebo-controlled, randomized trial. But that quickly went downhill when the researchers chose the type of magnesium to use in the trial. They chose magnesium oxide, the most poorly-absorbed form of magnesium commonly available (Moslehi, Vafa, Rahimi-Foroushani, & Golestan, 2012).[312] Tests show that the average human can only absorb 2–4 % of the magnesium in magnesium oxide, which makes it a great laxative, but a very poor supplement. That means that the 250 mg of magnesium oxide supplement that the subjects received each day during the trial, provided them with only about 5 to 10 mg of elemental magnesium that they could actually absorb, a negligible amount. So the resulting data were useless.

Now you and I are not the only ones in the world who are aware of the fact that magnesium oxide is the poorest possible choice for a magnesium supplement. So how is it possible that four supposedly qualified medical researchers were not aware of that fact? Did their medical training fail them? What went wrong with any peer reviews before the article was published that caused the reviewing physicians in charge of verifying the information to fail to notice the problem?

Here's an example of a research study that was doomed to be a waste of time and money right from the start.

This study involved re-analyzing the data from several large previous studies where information on the diets of the subjects was available. The goal of the project was obviously to prove that a plant-based diet was better than an animal-based diet for the health of the subjects in the study. And after a lot of complex mathematics, Satija et al (2016) showed that plant-based diets were indeed better for preventing type 2 diabetes than meat-based diets.[313] So why was the project doomed to reach a misleading conclusion right from the outset? Look at some of the food sources that contain the highest amounts of magnesium:

1. Dark leafy greens, such as spinach
2. Seeds, such as pumpkin seeds, and squash seeds
3. Beans and Lentils
4. Whole grains, such as brown rice
5. Fish, such as mackerel
6. Nuts, especially almonds
7. Dark Chocolate
8. Yogurt
9. Avocado
10. Banana

How many meats or animal-based foods do you see in that list? Precious few, to say the least. These are the types of food commonly found in larger quantities in plant-based diets, but they are usually present only in much smaller quantities in animal-based diets. We know from some of our previous discussions in this book (discussions that are well-referenced by research data) that magnesium deficiency is strongly associated with type 2 diabetes. So clearly, even though the researchers failed to acknowledge this association, and they did not measure (at least they did not report) magnesium levels of either the subjects in the study or their diets, this was actually a study of the effects of magnesium intake on the prevalence of type 2 diabetes.

So yes, the study may have verified the benefits of increased magnesium intake on the prevention of type 2 diabetes, but this hardly justifies going to all that trouble just so they could attribute it to a plant-based diet unless they had a preconceived agenda. And of course that preconceived agenda was to try to prove that a plant-based diet is better than an animal-based diet. But people following a plant-based diet still have a risk of developing diabetes (at a somewhat lower level) so the real message here is that virtually everyone should supplement their diet with extra magnesium if they want to prevent the development of type 2 diabetes. At any rate, failing to consider magnesium levels in this study is a scientifically-confounding factor that makes the results and conclusions c;aimed in the study mostly irrelevant.

Now the American Heart Association has joined the chorus, singing praises about the plant-based diet.

They've officially declared that eating a mostly plant-based diet can reduce the risk of developing heart failure by 42 %.[314] But again, this is misguided policy due to attributing the benefits of magnesium supplementation to a plant-based diet. That may be technically correct, but it is very misleading and it amounts to manipulating the facts in order to support the illusion that a meat-based diet might somehow be an unhealthy choice. As mentioned previously, normal amounts of vegetables no longer supply sufficient amounts of magnesium as they once did, because soils are becoming more depleted of magnesium. So the basic problem is depleted soils, not animal-based diets.

In an article written by researchers who have a vivid imagination, referring to certain species of gut microbes, the authors claim that "if you don't feed them, they can eat you".

Is this technical writing, or science fiction? You be the judge. The researchers began with mice that were free of gut bacteria (Lambert, & Vojdani, 2017).[315] Then they implanted 14 bacterial species so that they could follow the progress of the bacteria. They noted that bacteria that depend on fiber for survival, cannot survive normally on a low-fiber diet. So far, so good. Then they noted that in desperation, one of the species attempted to survive by ingesting mucus.

In the real world, survival of gut bacteria is determined by the rule of survival of the fittest. When a bacterial species is in survival mode, obviously it is not thriving. Gut bacteria that are not able to thrive in the gut are soon crowded out by other species that are able to thrive in the current environment associated with the current diet and digestive status. Gut bacteria that do not thrive, typically die, because they are unable to compete for space. They are not likely to "eat you", as speculated by the article, simply because they will not be around long enough to do that.

The bacterium claimed by the article to be capable of this contrived threat is Citrobacter rodentium. Have you ever heard of anyone who became ill because of an overgrowth of C. rodentium? The reason you have not is because C. rodentium is only found in the guts of mice (that fact is even noted in their name). So unless you or I have a mouse hidden somewhere in our family tree, we are not likely to have C. rodentium in our intestines.

Someone will surely point out that C. rodentium in mice is similar to E. coli in the human gut. True, this species is considered to be a murine (mouse-based) analogue used in studies of human colitis. But the claims made in the article regarding the dire consequences for humans go far beyond the limits of good science. The article appears to be mostly smoke-and-mirrors-based sensationalism, in an attempt to scare people. Note that the lead author is affiliated with Cyrex Laboratories. Cyrex Laboratories makes a lot of money from testing for human gut bacteria, parasites, and food allergies.

For years longevity experts have claimed that the key to living a long healthy life is to avoid saturated fats.

Since cardiovascular issues are the number one cause of death, many medical professionals have insisted that cholesterol levels determine the primary risks that are associated with longevity. But research disputes that claim. A recent study of old data (the Minnesota Coronary Experiment of 1968–1973) in which the subjects changed their diet by switching to corn oil, showed that the dietary switch from saturated fats did indeed lower cholesterol levels, but instead of living longer, they died sooner (Ramsden et al., 2016).[316] In fact, for every 30 mg/dl (0.78 mmol/l) reduction in total serum cholesterol, the risk of death increased by about 22 %.

The American Heart Association recently released an advisory warning that the use of saturated fats in the diet can lead to cardiovascular disease.

But this is basically a repeat of the same warning that they have been issuing for decades. And more than a few authorities have pointed out that similar to the previous warnings, it's based on flawed science. The report insists that replacing saturated fats in the diet with polyunsaturated vegetable oils will lead to approximately a 30 % reduction in cardiovascular disease (Sacks et al, 2017, June 15).[317] Saturated fats include animal-based fats and coconut oil, both of which have been shown by numerous research projects to reduce cardiovascular risk. But the very next day after this report was published, USA Today jumped on the bandwagon by publishing an article aimed at discrediting the use of coconut oil (May, 2017, June 16).[318]

An explanation of why this report is based on fake science requires a long and detailed account. If you are interested, the details are best explained by the investigative science and health journalist, Gary Taubes (Taubes, 2017, June 17).[319] Basically, according to Taubes, The American Heart Association threw out all the research that disagreed with their position and kept four arguably compromised studies that were done in the 1960s (which happened to agree with their position). All of the more recent research was rejected, and so was all the research studies that involved women subjects, resulting in a very biased report.

Before you decide how you will handle fats in your own diet, you should read some of the research reports that The American Heart Association chose to ignore, or at least read the conclusions stated in the reports. In 2010, for example, Siri-Tarino, Sun, Hu, and Krauss pointed out that the research concerning the association of the intake of saturat-

256

ed fats and cardiovascular disease has been inconsistent.[320]   In addition, replacing saturated fats with a higher carbohydrate intake, particularly refined carbohydrates, can increase insulin resistance, triglycerides, and obesity. It can also cause an increase in the level of small LDL particles, and a decrease in HDL cholesterol.

In 2016, Pimpin, Wu, Haskelberg, Del Gobbo, and Mozaffarian published evidence showing that when comparing all the available research, an animal fat product, butter, shows little to no association with cardiovascular disease, mortality, or diabetes.[321]

And in a huge study involving subjects in 18 countries from 5 continents, Dehghan et al. (2017) showed that total fat and individual types of fat were related to lower total mortality.[322] They also showed that total fat and types of fat were not associated with cardiovascular disease, myocardial infarction, or cardiovascular disease mortality. And they showed that high carbohydrate intake was associated with higher risk of total mortality. They even showed that higher saturated fat intakes were associated with reduced stroke risk. This study blows the position of The American Heart Association out of the water. Clearly, The American Heart Association does not appear to be interested in advocating good health practices based on medical science. It appears to be mainly interested in promoting it's own selfish and unscientific agenda.

To wrap up this section on misleading research, here's an example of a research article conclusion that's both dishonest and invalid.

A headline in the January 24, 2017 issue of the London Daily Express announced, "HEALTH WARNING: Just ONE cheeseburger or pizza binge 'could alter your metabolism", (Sheldrick, 2017, January 24).[323] The first line of the article stated, "A SINGLE cheeseburger or pizza blow-out can alter metabolism and trigger changes linked to fatty liver disease and diabetes, research has shown".

That sounds serious, and the article is based on a research report published in The Journal of Clinical Investigation (JCI), which is recognized as a peer-reviewed biomedical research journal published by the American Society for Clinical Investigation (ASCI) (Hernández et al., 2017).[324]

But further investigation reveals that both articles are based on data that are not only misleading, but they appear to be scientifically dishonest because of the corrupt methods used by the researchers. A quote taken from the Express article reveals the problem:

> *"The practical implication of this work is that the PO (palm oil) challenge used in this study most likely resembles the effects of ingestion of a meal rich in saturated fat, eg an eight-slice pepperoni pizza .. or a meal consisting of a 110g cheeseburger and a large portion of french [sic] fries .*

A glass of vanilla-flavored palm oil most certainly does not resemble either of the meals that it was claimed to simulate . . . not by any reasonable stretch of the imagination. While the palm oil does contain fat, it's a unique fat that can't be found in either pepperoni pizza or a cheeseburger and French fries.

In fact, according to research published in 2012 by Laugerette et al, when compared with some other common fats, palm oil is highly inflammatory due to it's propensity to promote increased inflammatory endotoxin transport.[325] It definitely is not a suitable substitute for the meals stated in the articles, unless the goal is to "stack the deck" in order to get the desired research results.

Their article lists 72 medical references, but it comes as no surprise that the research by Laugerette et al. is not included. It seems rather unlikely that out of all the researchers involved with this project, not a single one was aware of the research by Laugerette et al., and they all made the same "honest" mistake in choosing palm oil by mere coincidence. Shame on them for using dishonest methods.

For decades the medical community denied the existence of non-celiac gluten sensitivity.

But medical proof of non-celiac gluten sensitivity has been published (Uhde et al., 2016).[326] This study was the first to show that for a group of people who are not celiacs and are not allergic to wheat, but who still show clinical symptoms if they eat gluten, there are definite biological changes to their bodies triggered by exposure to gluten. The most important finding appears to be that for these individuals, exposure to gluten causes increased intestinal permeability, especially in the jejunum, which is the middle segment of the small intestine. And the increased permeability can subsequently cause food sensitivities. This results in basically the same clinical symptoms as celiac disease, including bloating, pain, diarrhea, fatigue, brain fog and other neurological symptoms. And while they may show inflammation of the villi of their small intestine upon biopsy examination under the microscope, they do not develop the complete villus atrophy that is the hallmark of celiac disease. It's thought that as many as 6 % of the general population may possibly have non-celiac gluten sensitivity, which if true, would mean that there may be about twice as many people with non celiac gluten sensitivity as there are celiacs.

But the medical community is so protective of what it considers to be it's own "turf" that it appears to be very resentful of anyone who dares to follow a GF diet without an official medical diagnosis of celiac disease.

As an example of how biased medical researchers tend to be concerning patients who follow a gluten-free diet without an official diagnosis, consider the following asinine study. In an apparent effort to coerce anyone who doesn't have an official celiac diagnosis, but who follows the GF diet anyway, into abandoning the diet, Zong et al. (2017, March 09) went to the trouble of showing that a celiac diet tends to increase the risk of type 2 diabetes.[327] This was (not surprisingly) presented at a March, 2017 meeting of the American Heart Association's Epidemiology and Prevention / Lifestyle and Cardiometabolic Health 2017 Scientific Sessions in Portland, Oregon.

The biggest problem with this "research" is that we already knew that diabetes is associated with gluten sensitivity (rather than the GF diet), and the main reason why most people follow the GF diet is because they are sensitive to gluten and they feel better when it is avoided, despite a negative celiac test result, and despite claims from the medical community that the GF diet is just a "fad" diet.

Shame on the medical community for trying to persuade people to eschew the GF diet, when in fact the GF diet makes them feel better and is likely to significantly improve their long-term health. If the medical community was actually interested in improving the health of patients, it would be promoting the GF diet, because avoiding gluten provides health benefits for almost everyone who follows it, whether or not they appear to react to gluten.

Why does mainstream medicine remain so out--of-touch with reality regarding non-celiac gluten sensitivity?

Could their feigned ignorance be intentional? Are they simply loathe to admit that they've been wrong about non-celiac gluten sensitivity for so many years? Here's just one example among many where researchers pretend that anyone who follows a gluten-free diet without an official diagnosis of celiac disease is guilty of deviant behavior. This attitude is the height of audacity in view of the fact that the mainstream medical community doesn't even have an approved method for diagnosing non-celiac gluten sensitivity. They expect their patients to continue to suffer so that the medical community can save face and maintain it's status of professional ignorance. And this is the apparent position of presumably the most prestigious medical institutions in the U. S, as illustrated by a paper from the Mayo Clinic (Choung et al., 2017).[328]

Dutch researchers have found that both the highest and lowest levels of magnesium can increase the probability of developing dementia.

In a study involving over 9,500 men and women, researchers found that people with either the highest or the lowest levels of magnesium in their blood had an increased risk of developing all-cause dementia, and the increased risk was as much as 30 % higher (Kieboom et al., 2017).[329] This was true for magnesium levels equal to or below 1.92 ng/ml (0.79 mmol/l), or equal to or above 2.19 ng/ml (0.90 mmol/l). Now the normal range usually used by most labs is 1.7–2.2 ng/ml (0.70–0.90 mmol/l), so while the high end of the normal range seems correct, the low end appears to be too low to prevent an increased dementia risk. Based on the dementia research results, the normal range used by labs for the serum magnesium test should actually be 1.9–2.2 ng/ml (0.76–0.90 nmol/l).

Fecal microbiota transplantation (FMT) has generated a lot of interest as a possible treatment for inflammatory bowel disease.

A systematic review and meta-analysis of eighteen past studies has been made by Colman and Rubin, (2014).[330] They concluded that FMT has highly variable results when used to treat IBD. In the overall analysis, among 79 ulcerative colitis patients, 39 Crohn's patients, and 4 unclassified IBD patients, FMT brought remission for 22 % of ulcerative colitis patients and 60.5 % of Crohn's patients. This was an overall success rate of 54 of 119 (45 %) patients. Due to the fact that followups were only for a very short time period, estimates of the average length of remission times are not available. Obviously this needs more research.

Research data on FMT treatments for microscopic colitis are lacking.

To date, there don't appear to be any published articles claiming success with FMT for treating microscopic colitis. There are case studies where recurring C. difficile was successfully treated in a patient who apparently then developed MC as a result of the recurring C. difficile, for example (Fasullo, Al-Azzawi, & Abergel, 2017, July 19).[331] There is also at least one case study that shows a new diagnosis of MC after an FMT attempt to treat UC (Tariq, Smyrk, Pardi, Tremaine, & Khanna, 2016).[332] But apparently, so far at least, attempts to treat MC with FMT have been generally unsuccessful.

The current status of microscopic colitis as viewed by many in the medical community.

For a very comprehensive discussion of the prevailing medical viewpoint on MC, this article published by the European Microscopic Colitis Group (EMCG) is probably one of the best (Münch et al., 2012).[333] This article not only discusses the disease itself, but it covers leaky gut, and accepted medical treatments. The statistics on the incidence of the disease, current diagnostic criteria, and drug associations are discussed. As might be expected, all the recommended treatments are drug or surgical-based, with no mention of food sensitivities or diet change recommendations.

Perhaps the most important research concerning the development of inflammatory bowel disease to be published in decades focuses on a series of minor food poisoning events that may cause cumulative damage that leads up to the development of IBD.

Yang et al. (2017) showed that relatively minor food poisoning events involving a very common bacteria, Salmonella Typhimurium, can lead to a series of events that culminate in the development of IBD.[334] The researchers showed that this can happen even when the infection is so mild that there are no significant symptoms and the Salmonella are easily eliminated by the immune system. In the study, four repeated infections were sufficient to cause the development of IBD.

Yang et al. (2017) noted that the Salmonella induced an acquired deficiency of intestinal alkaline phosphatase (IAP), an enzyme that is normally produced by the small intestine to remove phosphates from molecules such as the lipopolysaccharide (LPS) byproducts of various bacteria normally found in the colon. The IAP deficiency allows LPS to remain in a toxic, pro-inflammatory form.

This leads to a state of chronic inflammation that tends to be reinforced by repeated minor infections, and eventually the result is IBD. Perhaps in the future, IAP levels can be monitored, and if a deficiency is detected, it can be supplemented to prevent the development of IBD.

Summary

A huge volume of research has been published in recent years that is of interest to microscopic colitis patients. As usual, one has to look at most research articles these days with a critical eye because many of them may be misleading, and some appear to be downright dishonest. But all in all, researchers are making progress They may be getting close to finally being able to state with certainty just what causes microscopic colitis and other inflammatory bowel diseases. Once we know what actually causes a disease, we may be within reach of more effective ways to control it.

About the Author

Wayne Persky BSME

Wayne Persky was born, grew up, and currently lives in Central Texas. He is a graduate of the University of Texas at Austin, College of Engineering, with postgraduate studies in mechanical engineering, mathematics, and computer science. He has teaching experience in engineering, and business experience in farming and agribusiness.

After the onset of severe digestive system and general health problems in the late 1990s, he went through extensive clinical testing, but the GI specialist failed to take biopsies during a colonoscopy exam, and even failed to test for celiac disease. Afterward, not surprisingly, he was told by his gastroenterologist that there was nothing wrong with him.

Unable to find a medical solution, he was forced to use his research skills to discover innovative ways to resolve his health issues. After extensive study, he identified the likely source of the problem as food sensitivities triggered by the intestinal inflammation associated with inflammatory bowel disease.

It took a year and a half of avoiding all traces of gluten, plus trial and error experimentation with other foods, and careful record-keeping, to track down all of the food issues. But once he eliminated all of them from his diet, he got his life back. Over 15 years later, he continues to actively study new medical research as it becomes available. He currently administrates an online microscopic colitis discussion and support forum where valuable real world information about living with the disease and controlling the symptoms is shared world-wide. He also founded and participates in the Microscopic Colitis Foundation.

Contact Details:

Wayne Persky can be contacted at:
Persky Farms
19242 Darrs Creek Rd
Bartlett, TX 76511
USA

Tel: 1(254)718-1125
Tel: 1(254)527-3682

Email: wayne@microscopiccolitisfoundation.org
Email: wayne@waynepersky.com

For information and support regarding microscopic colitis, visit:

http://www.microscopiccolitisfoundation.org/

Participate in the Discussion and Support Forum:

http://www.perskyfarms.com/phpBB2/index.php

My author website can be found at waynepersky.com

Alphabetical Index

References

1 Persky, W. (2012). *Microscopic Colitis*. Bartlett, TX: Persky Farms.

2 Hamsten, C., Tran, T. A. T., Starkhammar, M., Brauner, A., Commins, S. P., Platts-Mills, T. A. E., & van Hage, M. (2013). Red meat allergy in Sweden: Association with tick sensitization and B-negative blood groups. *The Journal of Allergy and Clinical Immunology, 132*(6), 1431–1434. Retrieved from https://www.ncbi.nlm.nih.gov/pmc/articles/PMC4036066/

3 Nunen, S. (2015). Tick-induced allergies: mammalian meat allergy, tick anaphylaxis and their significance. *Asia Pacific Allergy, 5*(1), 3–16. Retrieved from https://www.ncbi.nlm.nih.gov/pmc/articles/PMC4313755/

4 Allergy Researchers. (n.d.). A resource on the mammalian meat allergy. *University of Virginia.* Retrieved from https://allergytomeat.wordpress.com/frequently-asked-questions/

5 Drago, S., El Asmar, R., Di Pierro, M., Grazia, C. M., Tripathi, A., Sapone, A., . . . Fasano, A. (2006). Gliadin, zonulin and gut permeability: Effects on celiac and non-celiac intestinal mucosa and intestinal cell lines. *Scandinavian Journal of Gastroenterology, 41*(4), 408–19. Retrieved from http://www.ncbi.nlm.nih.gov/pubmed/16635908

6 Fasano, A. (2012). Zonulin, regulation of tight junctions, and autoimmune diseases. *Annals of the New York Academy of Sciences, 1258*(1), 25–33. Retrieved from https://www.ncbi.nlm.nih.gov/pmc/articles/PMC3384703/

7 Uhde, M., Ajamian, M., Caio, G., De Giorgio, R., Indart, A., Green, P. H., . . . Alaedini, A. (2016). Intestinal cell damage and systemic immune activation in individuals reporting sensitivity to wheat in the

absence of coeliac disease. *Gut*, pii, gutjnl-2016-311964. Retrieved from http://gut.bmj.com/content/early/2016/07/21/gutjnl-2016-311964.full

8 Eades, M. (2006, August 30). Is increased fiber intake really a good thing? *The Blog of Michael R. Eades, M.D.* Retrieved from https://proteinpower.com/drmike/2006/08/30/is-increased-fiber-intake-really-a-good-thing/

9 Posadzki, P., Watson, L., & Ernst, E. (2013). Contamination and adulteration of herbal medicinal products (HMPs): an overview of systematic reviews. *The European Journal of Clinincal Pharmacology, 69*(3), 295-307. Retrieved from Eur J Clin Pharmacol. 2013 Mar;69(3):295-307. Retrieved from https://www.ncbi.nlm.nih.gov/pubmed/22843016

10 Harris, G. (2013, October 31). F.D.A. finds 12% of U.S. spice imports contaminated. *The New York Times*. p. A3. Retrieved from http://www.nytimes.com/2013/10/31/health/12-percent-of-us-spice-imports-contaminated-fda-finds.html

11 Bosma-den Boer, M. M., van Wetten, M.-L., & Pruimboom, L. (2012). Chronic inflammatory diseases are stimulated by current lifestyle: how diet, stress levels and medication prevent our body from recovering. *Nutrition & Metabolism, 9*(1), 32. Retrieved from https://www.ncbi.nlm.nih.gov/pmc/articles/PMC3372428/

12 Koskela, R. (2011). *Microscopic colitis: Clinical features and gastroduodenal and immunogenic findings.* (Doctoral dissertation, University of Oulu). Retrieved from http://herkules.oulu.fi/isbn9789514294150/isbn9789514294150.pdf

13 Pitchumoni, C. S., Rubin, A., & Das, K. (2010). Pancreatitis in inflammatory bowel diseases. *Journal of Clinical Gastroenterology, 44*(4), 246–253. Retrieved from https://www.ncbi.nlm.nih.gov/pubmed/20087199

14 Sullivan, K. (2016, October 5). The lectin report. *Krispin's Komments on Nutrition and Health.* Retrieved from http://www.krispin.com/lectin.html

15 Kolberg, J., & Sollid, L. (1985). Lectin activity of gluten identified as wheat germ agglutinin. *Biochemical and Biophysical Research Communications, 130*(2),867-72. Retrieved from https://www.ncbi.nlm.nih.gov/pubmed/3839672

16 Mercola, J. (2011, July 05). These five foods may cause problems very similar to wheat. *Mercola.com,* Retrieved from http://articles.mercola.com/sites/articles/archive/2011/07/05/other-nonwheat-grains-can-also-hurt-your-health.aspx

17 Lenardon, M. D., Munro, C. A., & Gow, N. A. R. (2010). Chitin synthesis and fungal pathogenesis. *Current Opinion in Microbiology, 13*(4), 416–423. Retrieved from https://www.ncbi.nlm.nih.gov/pmc/articles/PMC2923753/

18 Makowska, B., Bakera, B., & Rakoczy-Trojanowska, M. (2015). The genetic background of benzoxazinoid biosynthesis in cereals. *Acta Physiologiae Plantarum, 37*(1), 176. Retrieved from http://link.springer.com/article/10.1007/s11738-015-1927-3

19 Savelkoul, F. H., van der Poel, A.F., & Tamminga, S. (1992). The presence and inactivation of trypsin inhibitors, tannins, lectins and amylase inhibitors in legume seeds during germination. A review. *Plant Foods for Human Nutrition, 42*(1), 71-85. Retrieved from

https://www.ncbi.nlm.nih.gov/pubmed/1372122

20 Junker, Y., Zeissig, S., Kim, S.-J., Barisani, D., Wieser, H., Leffler, D. A., . . . Schuppan, D. (2012). Wheat amylase trypsin inhibitors drive intestinal inflammation via activation of toll-like receptor 4. *Journal of Experimental Medicine, 209*(13), 2395–2408. Retrieved from https://www.ncbi.nlm.nih.gov/pmc/articles/PMC3526354/

21 Guandalini, S. (2007, summer). A brief history of celiac disease. *Impact, The University of Chicago Celiac Disease Center. 7*(3). Retrieved from https://www.cureceliacdisease.org/wp-content/uploads/SU07CeliacCtr.News_.pdf

22 Li, X., Wang, C., Nie, J., Lv, D., Wang, T., & Xu, Y. (2013). Toll-like receptor 4 increases intestinal permeability through up-regulation of membrane PKC activity in alcoholic steatohepatitis. *Alcohol, 47*(6), 459–465. Retrieved from https://www.ncbi.nlm.nih.gov/pubmed/23871536

23 Oostenbrug, L. E., Drenth, J. P., de Jong, D.J., Nolte, I. M., Oosterom, E., van Dullemen, H. M., . . . Jansen, P. L. (2005). Association between Toll-like receptor 4 and inflammatory bowel disease. *Inflammatory Bowel Diseases, 11*(6), 567-575. Retrieved from https://www.ncbi.nlm.nih.gov/pubmed/15905704

24 Fukata, M., Shang, L., Santaolalla, R., Sotolongo, J., Cristhine Pastorini, C., España, C., . . . Abreu, M. T. (2011). Constitutive activation of epithelial TLR4 augments inflammatory responses to mucosal injury and drives colitis-associated tumorigenesis. *Inflammatory Bowel Diseases, 17*(7), 1464–1473. Retrieved from https://www.ncbi.nlm.nih.gov/pmc/articles/PMC3117047/

25 Unitt, J., & Hornigold, D. (2011). Plant lectins are novel Toll-like receptor agonists. *Biochemical Pharmacology, 81*(11), 1324-1328. Retrieved from https://www.ncbi.nlm.nih.gov/pubmed/21420389

26 Koller, B., Müller-Wiefel, A. S., Rupec, R., Korting, H. C., & Ruzicka, T. (2011). Chitin modulates innate immune responses of keratinocytes. *PLoS ONE 6*(2), e16594. Retrieved from http://journals.plos.org/plosone/article?id=10.1371/journal.pone.0016594

27 Dheer, R., Santaolalla, R., Davies, J. M., Lang, J. K., Phillips, M. C., Pastorini, C., . . . Abreu, M. T. (2016). Intestinal epithelial toll-like receptor 4 signaling affects epithelial function and colonic microbiota and promotes a risk for transmissible colitis. *Infection and Immunity, 84*(3), 798-810. Retrieved from http://iai.asm.org/content/84/3/798.full

28 Kressor, C, (n.d.). Beyond paleo. *Chris Kressor.* Retrieved from https://chriskresser.com/beyond-paleo-2/

29 Treatment by diet changes. (n.d.). *Microscopic Colitis Foundation.* Retrieved from http://www.microscopiccolitisfoundation.org/using-diet-changes.html

30 St-Onge, M.-P., Ard, J., Baskin, M. L., Chiuve, S. E., Johnson, H. M., Kris-Etherton, P., & Varady, K., On behalf of the American Heart Association Obesity Committee of the Council on Lifestyle and Cardiometabolic Health; Council on Cardiovascular Disease in the Young; Council on Clinical Cardiology; and Stroke Council. (2017, January 30). Meal timing and frequency: Implications for cardiovascular disease prevention: A scientific statement from the American Heart Association. *The American Heart Association.* Retrieved from http://circ.ahajournals.org/content/early/2017/01/30/CIR.0000000000000476.full.pdf?download=true

31 Mekary, R. A., Giovannucci, E., Willett, W. C., van Dam, R. M., & Hu, F. B. (2012). Eating patterns and type 2 diabetes risk in men: breakfast omission, eating frequency, and snacking. *American Journal of Clinical Nutrition, 95*(5), 1182-1189. Retrieved from http://ajcn.nutrition.org/content/95/5/1182.full

32 Mekary, R.A., Giovannucci, E., Cahill, L., Willett, W. C., van Dam, R. M., Hu, F. B. (2013). Eating patterns and type 2 diabetes risk in older women: breakfast consumption and eating frequency. *American Journal of Clinical Nutrition 98*(1), 436–443. Retrieved fromhttps://www.ncbi.nlm.nih.gov/pmc/articles/PMC3712552/

33 Uemura, M., Yatsuya, H., Hilawe, E. H., Li, Y., Wang, C., Chiang, C. . . . Otsuka,R. (2015). Breakfast skipping is positively associated with incidence of type 2 diabetes mellitus: evidence from the Aichi Workers' Cohort Study. *International Journal of Epidemiology, 25*(1), 351–358. Retrieved from https://www.ncbi.nlm.nih.gov/pmc/articles/PMC4411234/

34 Odegaard, A.O., Jacobs, D. R. Jr., Steffen, L. M., Van Horn, L., Ludwig, D. S., & Pereira, M. A. (2013). Breakfast frequency and development of metabolic risk. *Diabetes Care. 36*(1), 3100–3106. Retrieved from http://care.diabetesjournals.org/content/36/10/3100.long

35 Mozes, A. (2017, August 3). Protein at all 3 meals may help preseerve senior's strength. Retrieved from https://consumer.healthday.com/senior-citizen-information-31/misc-aging-news-10/protein-at-all-3-meals-may-help-preserve-seniors-strength-725178.html

36 Horne, B. D., Muhlestein, J. B., May, H. T., Carlquist, J. F., Lappé, D. L., Bair, T. L., . . . Intermountain Heart Collaborative Study Group. (2012). Relation of routine, periodic fasting to risk of diabetes melli-

tus, and coronary artery disease in patients undergoing coronary angiography. *American Journal of Cardiology,109*(11), 1558-1562. Retrieved from http://www.ajconline.org/article/S0002-9149%2812%2900595-4/abstract

37 Ma, Y., Bertone, E. R., Stanek, E. J. 3rd, Reed, G.W., Hebert, J. R., Cohen, N. L., . . . Ockene, I. S. (2003). Association between eating patterns and obesity in a free-living US adult population. *American Jourtnal of Epidemiology, 158*(1), 85-92 Retrieved from https://www.ncbi.nlm.nih.gov/pubmed/12835290

38 Holmbäck, I., Ericson, U., Gullberg, B., & Wirfält, E. (2010). A high eating frequency is associated with an overall healthy lifestyle in middle-aged men and women and reduced likelihood of general and central obesity in men. *British Journal of Nutrition, 104*(7), 1065–1073. Retrieved from https://www.ncbi.nlm.nih.gov/pubmed/20500929

39 Harvie, M. N., Pegington, M., Mattson, M. P., Frystyk, J., Dillon, B., Evans, G., . . . Howell, A. (2011). The effects of intermittent or continuous energy restriction on weight loss and metabolic disease risk markers: a randomized trial in young overweight women. *International Journal of Obesity, 35*(5), 714–727. Retrieved from https://www.ncbi.nlm.nih.gov/pubmed/20921964

40 Heilbronn, L. K., Smith, S. R., Martin, C. K., Anton, S. D., & Ravussin, E.(2005). Alternate-day fasting in nonobese subjects: effects on body weight, body composition, and energy metabolism. *American Journal of Clinical Nutrition 81*(1), 69-73. Retrieved from http://ajcn.nutrition.org/content/81/1/69.full

41 Eshghinia, S, & Mohammadzadeh, F. (2013). The effects of modified alternate-day fasting diet on weight loss and CAD risk factors in

overweight and obese women. *Journal of Diabetes & Metabolic Disorders.*12(1), 4. Retrieved from
https://www.ncbi.nlm.nih.gov/pubmed/23497604

42 Johnson, J. B., Summer, W., Cutler, R. G., Martin, B., Hyun, D. H., Dixit, V. D., . . . Mattson, M. P. (2007). Alternate day calorie restriction improves clinical findings and reduces markers of oxidative stress and inflammation in overweight adults with moderate asthma. *Free Radical Biology & Medicine.* 42(5), 665–674. Retrieved from
https://www.ncbi.nlm.nih.gov/pubmed/17291990

43 Varady, K. A., Bhutani, S, Church, E. C., & Klempel, M. C. (2009). Short-term modified alternate-day fasting: a novel dietary strategy for weight loss and cardioprotection in obese adults. *American Journal Clinical of Nutrition, 90*(5), 1138–1143. Retrieved from
https://www.ncbi.nlm.nih.gov/pubmed/19793855

44 Klempel, M. C., Kroeger, C. M., & Varady, K. A. (2013). Alternate day fasting (ADF) with a high-fat diet produces similar weight loss and cardio-protection as ADF with a low-fat diet. *Metabolism, 62*(1), 137–143. Retrivied from https://www.ncbi.nlm.nih.gov/pubmed/22889512

45 Hoddy, K. K., Kroeger, C. M., Trepanowski, J. F., Barnosky, A., Bhutani, S., & Varady, K. A. (2014). Meal timing during alternate day fasting: Impact on body weight and cardiovascular disease risk in obese adults. *Obesity, 22*(12), 2524–2531. Retrieved from
https://www.ncbi.nlm.nih.gov/pubmed/25251676

46 Bhutani, S., Klempel, M. C., Kroeger, C. M., Trepanowski, J. F., & Varady, K. A. (2013). Alternate day fasting and endurance exercise combine to reduce body weight and favorably alter plasma lipids in obese humans. *Obesity, 21*(7), 1370–1379. Retrieved from

https://www.ncbi.nlm.nih.gov/pubmed/23408502

47 Varady, K. A., Bhutani, S., Klempel, M. C., Kroeger, C. M., Trepanowski, J. F., Haus, J.M., . . . Calvo, Y. (2013). Alternate day fasting for weight loss in normal weight and overweight subjects: a randomized controlled trial. *Nutrition Journal, 12*(1), 146. Retrieved from https://www.ncbi.nlm.nih.gov/pubmed/24215592

48 Klempel, M. C., Kroeger, C. M., Bhutani, S., Trepanowski, J. F., & Varady, K. A. (2012). Intermittent fasting combined with calorie restriction is effective for weight loss and cardio-protection in obese women. *Nutrition Journal, 11*(1), 98. Retrieved from https://www.ncbi.nlm.nih.gov/pubmed/23171320

49 Goldsmith, P., McGarity, B., Walls, A., F., Church, M., K., Millward-Sadler, G. H., & Robertson, D. A. (1990). Corticosteroid treatment reduces mast cell numbers in inflammatory bowel disease. *Digestive Diseases and Sciences, 35*(11), 1409–1413. Retrieved from http://www.ncbi.nlm.nih.gov/pubmed/1977567

50 Hidalgo, A. A., Deeb, K. K., Pike, J. W., Johnson, C. S., & Trump, D. L. (2011). Dexamethasone enhances 1α,25-dihydroxyvitamin D3 effects by increasing vitamin D receptor transcription. *The Journal of Biological Chemistry, 286*, 36,228–36,237. Retrieved from https://www.ncbi.nlm.nih.gov/pmc/articles/PMC3196110/

51 Persky , W. (2014). *Vitamin D and Autoimmune Disease.* Bartlett, TX: Persky Farms

52 Lucendo, A. J. (2017). Drug exposure and the risk of microscopic colitis: A critical update. *Drugs in R & D, 17*(1) 79–89. Retrieved from https://link.springer.com/article/10.1007/s40268-016-0171-7

53 Koskela, R. (2011). *Microscopic colitis: Clinical features and gastroduodenal and immunogenic findings.* (Doctoral dissertation: University of Oulu). Retrieved from http://herkules.oulu.fi/isbn9789514294150/isbn9789514294150.pdf

54 Simondi, D., Pellicano, R., Reggiani, S., Pallavicino, F., David, E., Sguazzini, C., . . . Astegiano, M. (2010). A retrospective study on a cohort of patients with lymphocytic colitis. *Spanish Journal of Gastroenterology, 102*(6), 381–384. Retrieved from http://www.ncbi.nlm.nih.gov/pubmed/20575599

55 Wolber, R., Owen, D., & Freeman, H. (1990). Colonic lymphocytosis in patients with celiac sprue. *Human Pathology, 21*(11), 10921096. Retrieved from http://www.ncbi.nlm.nih.gov/pubmed/2227917

56 Fine, K. D., Lee, E. L., & Meyer, R. L. (1998). Colonic histopathology in untreated celiac sprue or refractory sprue: is it lymphocytic colitis or colonic lymphocytosis? *Human Pathology, 29*(12), 14331440. Retrieved from http://www.ncbi.nlm.nih.gov/pubmed/9865829

57 Barratt, S. M., Leeds, J. S., & Sanders, D. S. (2011). Quality of life in Coeliac Disease is determined by perceived degree of difficulty adhering to a gluten-free diet, not the level of dietary adherence ultimately achieved. *Journal of Gastrointestinal And Liver Diseases, 20*(3), 241–245. Retrieved from https://www.ncbi.nlm.nih.gov/pubmed/21961090

58 Matoori, S., Fuhrmann, G., & Leroux, J. C. (2013). Celiac disease: a challenging disease for pharmaceutical scientists. *Pharmaceutical Research, 30*(3), 619–626. Retrieved from https://www.ncbi.nlm.nih.gov/pubmed/23229860

59 Barta, Z., Toth, L., Szabo, G. G., &Szegedi, G. (2003). Collagenous colitis: constipation or diarrhoea? *Gut, 52*(8), 1230. Retrieved from https://www.ncbi.nlm.nih.gov/pmc/articles/PMC1773752/#!

60 Hadjivassiliou, M., Chattopadhyay, A. K., Davies-Jones, G. A. B., Gibson, A., Grünewald, R. A., & Lobo, A. J. (1997). Neuromuscular disorder as a presenting feature of coeliac disease. *Journal of Neurology, Neurosurgery, & Psychiatry, 63*, 770–775. Retrieved from http://jnnp.bmj.com/content/63/6/770.full

61 Hadjivassiliou, M., Grünewald, R. A., & Davies-Jones, G. A. B. (2002). Gluten sensitivity as a neurological illness. *Journal of Neurology, Neurosurgery, & Psychiatry, 72*(1), 560–563. Retrieved from http://jnnp.bmj.com/content/72/5/560.full

62 Abrams, J. A., Diamond, B., Rotterdam, H., & Green, P. H. (2004). Seronegative celiac disease: increased prevalence with lesser degrees of villous atrophy. *Digestive Diseases and Sciences, 49*(4), 546–550. Retrieved from http://www.ncbi.nlm.nih.gov/pubmed/15185855

63 Stefansson, V. (1935, December). Eskimos prove an all-meat diet provides excellent health. *Harper's Monthly Magazine.* Retrieved from http://www.biblelife.org/stefansson2.htm

64 Treatment by diet changes. (2017). *The Microscopic Colitis Foundation.* Retrieved from http://www.microscopiccolitisfoundation.org/using-diet-changes.html

65 Nguyen, G. C., Smalley, W. E., Vege, S. S., Carrasco-Labra, A., & the Clinical Guidelines Committee. (2016). American Gastroenterological Association Institute guideline on the medical management of microscopic colitis. *Gastroenterology, 150*, 242–246 Retrieved from

http://www.gastrojournal.org/article/S0016-5085%2815%2901625-X/pdf

66 Masclee, G. M., Coloma, P. M, Kuipers, E. J., & Sturkenboom, M., C. (2015). Increased risk of microscopic colitis with use of proton pump inhibitors and non-steroidal anti-inflammatory drugs. *American Journal of Gastroenterology, 110*(5), 749–759. Retrieved from https://www.ncbi.nlm.nih.gov/pubmed/25916221

67 Peña, A. S., & Rodrigo, L. (2015). Celiac disease and non-celiac gluten sensitivity. *OmniaScience*. Retrieved from http://omniascience.com/monographs/index.php/monograficos/article/download/223/136

68 Dicke, W. K., Weijrs, H. A., Van De Kamer, J. H. (1953).Coeliac disease. II. The presence in wheat of a factor having a deleterious effect in cases of coeliac disease. *Acta Paediatrica Scandinavica. 42*(1), 34–42. Retrieved from https://www.ncbi.nlm.nih.gov/pubmed/13050382

69 Anderson, C. M., Frazer, A. C., French, J. M., Hawkins, C. F., Ross, C. A. C., & Sammons, H. G. (1954). The influence of gluten and antibacterial agents on fat absorption in the sprue syndrome. *Gastroenterologia, 81*, 98–103.Retrieved from https://www.karger.com/Article/Pdf/199985

70 Cornell Food & Brand Lab, (2015, November 24). Consumers' response to food safety risks are altered due to prior commitment and preference. Medical Xpress. Reteieved from https://medicalxpress.com/news/2015-11-consumers-response-food-safety-due.html

71 A food labeling guide. (2013). *Food and Drug Administration: U. S. Department of Health and Human Services*. Retrieved from https://www.f-

da.gov/downloads/food/guidanceregulation/ucm265446.pdf

72 CFR - Code of Federal Regulations Title 21. (2016, September 9). *U. S. Food & Drug Administration.* Retreived from https://www.accessdata.f-da.gov/scripts/cdrh/cfdocs/cfcfr/cfrsearch.cfm?fr=501.22

73 Moyad, M. A., Brumfield, S. K., &Pienta, K. J. (1999). Vitamin E, alpha- and gamma-tocopherol, and prostate cancer. *Seminars in Urologic Oncology. 17*(2), 85–90. Retrieved from https://www.ncbi.nlm.nih.gov/pubmed/10332921

74 Jiang, Q., Christen, S., Shigenaga, M. K., & Ames, B. N. (2001). Gamma-Tocopherol, the major form of vitamin E in the US diet, deserves more attention. *American Journal of Clininical Nutrition, 74*(6) 714–722. Retrieved from http://ajcn.nutrition.org/content/74/6/714.long

75 Miyake, K., Tanaka, T., & McNeil, P. L. (2006). Disruption-induced mucus secretion: Repair and protection. *PLoS Biology, 4*(9), Retrieved from https://www.ncbi.nlm.nih.gov/pmc/articles/PMC1544361/

76 Underwood, J. (2006). The path to digestion is paved with repair. *PLoS Biology, 4*(9), Retrieved from https://www.ncbi.nlm.nih.gov/pmc/articles/PMC1551928/

77 Thompson, T., Lee, A. R., Grace, T. (2010). Gluten contamination of grains, seeds, and flours in the United States: a pilot study. *Journal of the American Dietetic Association. 110*(6), 937–940. Retrieved from https://www.ncbi.nlm.nih.gov/pubmed/20497786

78 Cross-reactivity. (n.d.). *The American Academy of Allergy, Asthma & Immunology.* Retrieved from https://www.aaaai.org/conditions-and-treatments/conditions-dictionary/cross-reactivity

79 Mayo Clinic staff. (2017). Food allergy *Mayo Foundation for Medical Education and Researc.h* Retrieved from http://www.mayoclinic.org/diseases-conditions/food-allergy/symp-toms-causes/dxc-20317255

80 Myers, A. (n.d.). 6 foods your body thinks are gluten. *Amy Mayers MD*. Retrieved from https://www.amymyersmd.com/2017/06/gluten-cross-reactivity/

81 Palmer, B. (2014, April 14). Allergies are the real midlife crisis. *Slate* Retrieved from http://www.slate.com/articles/health_and_science/medical_examiner/2014/04/allergy_in_children_and_adults_why_do_allergies_get_better_or_worse_at_certain.html

82 Smith, G. (2014, March 18). Those who outgrow food allergy can risk EoE. *Allergic Living*. Retrieved from https://allergicliving.com/2014/03/18/those-who-outgrow-food-allergy-can-risk-eoe/

83 NDTV Food Desk. (Updated: 2017, April 11). What makes extra-virgin olive oil healthier than the regular one? *NDTV*. Retrieved from http://food.ndtv.com/health/what-makes-extra-virgin-olive-oil-healthier-than-the-regular-one-1679976

84 The 14 fake olive oil companies are revealed now – Avoid these brands. (2017, February 13). Retrieved from http://natural-cureshouse.com/the-14-fake-olive-oil-companies-are-revealed-now-avoid-these-brands/

85 Sonnenburg, E., & Sonnenburg, J. (2016, February 25). The extinction inside our guts. *The Los Angeles Times: Opinion section*. Retrieved from

http://www.latimes.com/opinion/op-ed/la-oe-0225-sonnen-burg-gut-bacteria-extinction-20160225-story.html?utm_source=Newsletter&utm_medium=Click&utm_campaign=1428

86 Kristensen, N. B., Bryrup, T., Allin, K. H., Nielsen, T., Hansen, T.H., & Pedersen, O. (2010). Alterations in fecal microbiota composition by probiotic supplementation in healthy adults: a systematic review of randomized controlled trials. *Genome Medicine 8*, 52. Retrieved from https://genomemedicine.biomedcentral.com/articles/10.1186/s13073-016-0300-5

87 Ma, J., Folsom, A. R., Melnick, S. L., Eckfeldt, J. H., Sharrett, A. R., Nabulsi, A. A., . . . Metcalf, P. A. (1995). Associations of serum and dietary magnesium with cardiovascular disease, hypertension, diabetes, insulin, and carotid arterial wall thickness: the ARIC study. Atherosclerosis Risk in Communities Study. *Journal of Clinical Epidemiology, 48*(7), 927–940. Retrieved from https://www.ncbi.nlm.nih.gov/pubmed/7782801

88 Sircus, M. (2009, December 8). Magnesium deficiency symptoms and diagnosis. *DrSircus.com*. Retrieved from http://drsircus.com/magnesium/magnesium-deficiency-symptoms-diagnosis/

89 Magnesium. (updated 2016, February 11). National Institutes of Health. Retrieved from https://ods.od.nih.gov/factsheets/Magnesium-HealthProfessional/

90 Kiefer, D. (2007, February). Is your bottled water killing you? *Life Extension Magazine*. Retrieved from http://www.lifeextension.com/magazine/2007/2/report_water/Page-01

91 The history of water filters. (n.d.). *Historyofwaterfilters.com*. Retrieved from http://www.historyofwaterfilters.com/

92 Azoulay, A., Garzon, P. & Eisenberg, M. J. (2001). Comparison of the mineral content of tap water and bottled waters. *Journal of General Internal Medicine, 16*(3), 168–175. Retrieved from https://www.ncbi.nlm.nih.gov/pmc/articles/PMC1495189/

93 Liebscher D. H., & Liebscher, D. E. (2004). About the misdiagnosis of magnesium deficiency. *The Journal of the American College of Nutrition, 23*(6), 730S–731S. Retrieved from https://www.ncbi.nlm.nih.gov/pubmed/15637222

94 Touyz, R. M. (2004). Magnesium in clinical medicine. *Frontiers in Bioscience, 1*(9), 1278–1293. Retrieved from https://www.ncbi.nlm.nih.gov/pubmed/14977544

95 Deans, E. (2012, September 11). Is fibromyalgia due to a mineral deficiency? *Psychology Today*. Retrieved from https://www.psychologytoday.com/blog/evolutionary-psychiatry/201209/is-fibromyalgia-due-mineral-deficiency

96 Engen, D. J., McAllister, S. J., Whipple, M. O., Cha, S. S., Dion, L. J., Vincent, A., . . . Wahner-Roedler, D. L. (2015). Effects of transdermal magnesium chloride on quality of life for patients with fibromyalgia: a feasibility study. *Journal of Integrative Medicine, 13*(5), 306–313. Retrieved from http://www.jcimjournal.com/jim/FullText2.aspx?articleID=S2095-4964%2815%2960195-9

97 Fischer, K. Why it matters whether you're getting enough magnesium. (2917, September 21). Retrieved from http://www.sheknows.com/health-and-wellness/articles/1009485/more-magnesium-for-hor-

monal-balance

98 Advantages of magnesium bisglycinate chelate buffered. (n.d.). *Albion Laboratories, Inc.* Retrieved from http://www.albionminerals.com/human-nutrition/magnesium-white-paper

99 Cojocaru, I. M., Cojocaru, M., Tănăsescu, R., Iacob, S. A., & Iliescu, I. (2009). Changes of magnesium serum levels in patients with acute ischemic stroke and acute infections. *Romanian Journal of Internal Medicine, 47*(2), 169–671. Retrieved from https://www.ncbi.nlm.nih.-gov/pubmed/20067167

100King, D. E., Mainous, A. G. 3rd, Geesey, M. E., & Woolson, R. F. (2005).Dietary magnesium and C-reactive protein levels. *Journal of the American College of Nutrition, 24*(3), 166–171. Retrieved from https://www.ncbi.nlm.nih.gov/pubmed/15930481

101King, D. E., Mainous, A. G. 3rd., Geesey, M. E., Egan, B. M., & Rehman, S. (2006). Magnesium supplement intake and C-reactive protein levels in adults. *Nutrition Research, 26*(2006), 193–196. Retrieved from http://www.anaboliclabs.com/User/Document/Articles/Magnesium/6.%20King,%20MAGnesium,%202006.pdf

102FDA Drug Safety Communication: Low magnesium levels can be associated with long-term use of Proton Pump Inhibitor drugs (PPIs). (2016, April 07). Retrieved from https://www.fda.gov/Drugs/DrugSafety/ucm245011.htm

103Disease incidence prevention by serum 25(OH)D level. (2010, March 23). *GrassRootsHealth.* Retrieved from http://www.grassroot-

shealth.net/media/download/disease_incidence_prev_chart_032310.p
df

104Larsen, H. R. (n.d.). Magnesiun. The AFIB Report. Retrieved from
http://www.afibbers.org/magnesium.html

105Ashley (2012, Februaruy 10). How Much Magnesium Do I Need? Retrieved from http://www.ancient-minerals.com/blog-post/how-much-
magnesium/

106Massey, P. B. (2015, February 7). Magnesium can lower cholesterol,
studies show. *Daily Herald*. Retrieved from http://www.dailyherald.-
com/article/20150207/entlife/150209666/

107Rayssiguier, Y., Gueux, E., & Weiser, D. (1981). Effect of magnesium
deficiency on lipid metabolism in rats fed a high carbohydrate diet.
Journal of Nutrition, 111(11),1876–1883. Retrieved from
https://www.ncbi.nlm.nih.gov/pubmed/7299488

108Olatunji, L. A., & Soladoye, A. O. (2007). Effect of increased magnesium intake on plasma cholesterol, triglyceride and oxidative stress
in alloxan-diabetic rats. *African Journal of Mededicine and Medical Sciences, 36*(2), 155-161. Retrieved from
https://www.ncbi.nlm.nih.gov/pubmed/19205579

109Guerrero-Romero, F., & Rodríguez-Morán, M. (2000). Hypomagne-
semia is linked to low serum HDL-cholesterol irrespective of serum
glucose values. *Journal of Diabetes and its Complications, 14*(5), 272—
276. Retrieved from https://www.ncbi.nlm.nih.gov/pubmed/11113690

110Efstratiadis, G., Sarigianni, M., & Gougourelas, I. (2006). Hypomag-
nesemia and cardiovascular system. *Hippokratia, 10*(4), 147–152. Re-

trieved from https://www.ncbi.nlm.nih.gov/pmc/articles/PM-C2464251/

111 Eby, G. A. & Eby, K. L. (2006). Rapid recovery from major depression using magnesium treatment. *Medical Hypotheses, 67*(2), 362–370. Retrieved from http://www.medical-hypotheses.com/article/S0306-9877%2806%2900103-4/abstract?cc=y=

112Pattyn, T., Van Den Eede, F., Vanneste, S., Cassiers, L., Veltman, D. J., Van De Heyning, P., & Sabbe, B. C. (2016). Tinnitus and anxiety disorders: A review. *Hearing Research, 333*, 255–265. Retrieved from https://www.ncbi.nlm.nih.gov/pubmed/26342399

113Mercola, J. (2017, April 05). Can Magnesium Relieve Your Tinnitus? Retrieved from http://articles.mercola.com/sites/articles/archive/2017/04/05/magnesium-tinnitus-relief.aspx

114Kent, L. T. (2015, November 11). Hashimoto's and magnesium deficiency. *Livestrong.com*. Retrieved from http://www.livestrong.com/article/547017-hashimotos-and-magnesium-deficiency/

115Keefer, A. (2017, October 3). What beverages are high in magnesium and phosphorus? Retrieved from https://www.livestrong.com/article/529466-what-beverages-are-high--in-magnesium-and-phosphorus/

116Magnesium. (2015, August 06). University of Maryland Medical Center (UMMC). Retrieved from http://www.umm.edu/health/medical/altmed/supplement/magnesium

117Reddy, V., & Sivakumar, B. (1974). Magnesium-dependent vitamin-D-resistant rickets. *The Lancet, 303*(7864), 963–965. Retrieved from http://www.thelancet.com/journals/lancet/article/PIIS0140-6736%2874%2991265-3/abstract

118Rude, R. K., Adams, J. S., Ryzen, E., Endres, D. B., Niimi, H., Horst, R. L., . . . Singer, F. R. (1985). Low serum concentrations of 1,25-dihydroxyvitamin D in human magnesium deficiency. *The Journal of Clinical Endocrinology & Metabolism, 61*(5), 933–940. Retrieved from https://www.ncbi.nlm.nih.gov/pubmed/3840173

119Sircus, M. (2010, September 20). Dehydration. symptoms, causes and treatments. *DrSircus.com*. Retrieved from http://drsircus.com/water/dehydration-symptoms-causes-treatments/

120Pfotenhauer, K. M., & Shubrook, J. H. (2017). Vitamin D deficiency, its role in health and disease, and current supplementation recommendations. *The Journal of the American Osteopathic Association, 117*(5), 301-305. Retrieved from http://jaoa.org/article.aspx?articleid=2625276

121National Health and Nutrition Examination Survey. (2013, September 30). *Centers for Disease Control and Prevention*. Retrieved from https://www.cdc.gov/nchs/nhanes/index.htm

122Ginde, A. A., Liu, M. C., & Camargo Jr, C. A. (2009). Demographic differences and trends of vitamin D insufficiency in the US population, 1988-2004. *Archives of Internal Medicine, 169*(6), 626-632. Retrieved from http://jamanetwork.com/journals/jamainternalmedicine/fullarticle/414878

123Study: More than half of college football athletes have inadequate levels of vitamin D - Deficiency linked to muscle injuries. (2017,

March 16). *Hospital for Special Surgery: PR Newswire*. Retrieved from http://www.prnewswire.com/news-releases/study-more-than-half-of-college-football-athletes-have-inadequate-levels-of-vitamin-d---deficiency-linked-to-muscle-injuries-300422304.html

124Chemical exposure linked to lower vitamin D levels. (2016, September 20). *ScienceDaily*. Retrieved from https://www.sciencedaily.com/releases/2016/09/160920130828.htm

125Johns, L. E., Ferguson, K. K., & Meeker, J. D. (2016). Relationships Between Urinary Phthalate Metabolite and Bisphenol A Concentrations and Vitamin D Levels in U.S. Adults: National Health and Nutrition Examination Survey (NHANES), 2005–2010. *The Journal of Clinical Endocrinology & Metababolism 101*(11), 4062-4069. Retrieved from https://academic.oup.com/jcem/article-abstract/101/11/4062/2764946/Relationships-Between-Urinary-Phthalate-Metabolite?redirectedFrom=fulltext

126Vitamin D and your health: Breaking old rules, raising new hopes. (2007, February). Harvard Health Publications: *Harvard Medical School*. Retrieved from http://www.health.harvard.edu/newsletter_article/vitamin-d-and-your-health-breaking-old-rules-raising-new-hopes

127Tripkovic, L., Lambert, H., Hart, K., Smith, C. P., Bucca, G., Penson, S., . . . Lanham-New, S. (2012). Comparison of vitamin D2 and vitamin D3 supplementation in raising serum 25-hydroxyvitamin D status: a systematic review and meta-analysis1,2,3. *The American Journal of Clinical Nutrition, 95*(6), 1357–1364. Retrieved from https://www.ncbi.nlm.nih.gov/pmc/articles/PMC3349454/

128Group, E. (2014, June 9). Vitamin D3 vs. vitamin D2 – What's the difference? *Global Healing Center*. Retrieved from https://www.global-healingcenter.com/natural-health/vitamin-d3-vs-vitamin-d2/

129Takaya, J., Higashino, H., & Kobayashi, Y. (2004). Intracellular magnesium and insulin resistance. *Magnesium Research, 17*(2), 126-136. Retrieved from http://www.ncbi.nlm.nih.gov/pubmed/15319146

130Sircus, M. (2009, December 8). Reversing insulin resistance — The insulin magnesium story. *DrSircus.com*. Retrieved from http://drsircus.-com/diabetes/reversing-insulin-resistance-the-insulin-magnesium-story/

131Dean, C. (2012, August 15). Magnesium Is Crucial for Bones. Huffpost: *The Huffington Post.com*. Retrieved from http://www.huffington-post.com/carolyn-dean-md-nd/bone-health_b_1540931.html

132Li, K., Kaaks, R., Linseisen, J., & Rohrmann, S. (2012). Associations of dietary calcium intake and calcium supplementation with myocardial infarction and stroke risk and overall cardiovascular mortality in the Heidelberg cohort of the European Prospective Investigation into Cancer and Nutrition study (EPIC-Heidelberg) *Heart, 98*(12), 920-925. Retrieved from http://heart.bmj.com/content/98/12/920.full

133Kressor, C. (2013, March 8). Calcium supplements: Why you should think twice. *CrisKressor.com*. Retrieved from https://chriskresser.com/calcium-supplements-why-you-should-think-twice/

134Raftery, T., Martineau, A. R., Greiller, C. L., Ghosh, S., McNamara, D., Bennett, K., . . .O'Sullivan, M. (2015). Effects of vitamin D supplementation on intestinal permeability, cathelicidin and disease markers in Crohn's disease: Results from a randomised double-blind placebo-controlled study. *United European Gastroenterology Journal, 3*(3), 294–302. Retrieved from https://www.ncbi.nlm.nih.gov/pmc/articles/PMC4480538/

135Narula, N., Cooray, M., Anglin, R., & Marshall, J. (2017). Impact of high dose vitamin D3 supplementation in treatment of Crohn's disease in remission: A randomized double-blind controlled study. Digital diseases and Sciences, 62(2), 448–445. Retrieved from https://link.springer.com/article/10.1007/s10620-016-4396-7

136Kwon, K. Y., Jo, K. D., Lee, M. K., Oh, M, Kim, E. N., Park, J.,. . . . Jang, W. (2016). Low serum vitamin D levels may contribute to gastric dysmotility in de novo Parkinson's disease. *Neurodegenerative Diseases, 16*(3-4),199-205. Retrieved from https://www.ncbi.nlm.nih.gov/pubmed/26735311

137Mokry, L. E., Ross, S., Morris, J. A., Manousaki, D., Forgetta, V., & Richards, J. B. (2016). Genetically decreased vitamin D and risk of Alzheimer disease. *Neurology. 87*(24), 2567-2574. Retrieved from https://www.ncbi.nlm.nih.gov/pubmed/27856775

138Gubatan, J., Mitsuhashi, S., Zenlea, T., Rosenberg, L., Robson, S., & Moss, A. C. (2017). Low serum vitamin D during remission increases risk of clinical relapse in patients with ulcerative colitis. *Clinical Gastroenterology and Hepatology 15*(2), 240-246. Retrieved from https://www.ncbi.nlm.nih.gov/pubmed/27266980

139Winter, R. W., Collins, E., Cao, B., Carrellas, M., Crowell, A. M., & Korzenik, J. R. (2017). Higher 25-hydroxyvitamin D levels are associated with greater odds of remission with anti-tumour necrosis factor-α medications among patients with inflammatory bowel diseases. *Al-*

imentary Pharmacology and Theraputics, 45(5):653–659. Retrieved from
https://www.ncbi.nlm.nih.gov/pubmed/28074487

140Faridi, K. F., Zhao, D., Martin, S.S., Lupton, J. R., Jones, S, R., Guallar,
E., . . . Michos, E. D. (2017). Serum vitamin D and change in lipid levels over 5 y: The Atherosclerosis Risk in Communities study. *Nutrition, 38*(June), 85–93. Retrieved from http://www.nutritionjrnl.com/article/S0899-9007%2817%2930021-7/fulltext

141Asano, L., Watanabe, M., Ryoden, Y., Usuda, K., Yamaguchi, T.,
Khambu, B., . . . Uesugi, M. (2017). Vitamin D Metabolite, 25-Hydroxyvitamin D, Regulates Lipid Metabolism by Inducing Degradation of SREBP/SCAP. *Cell Chemical Biology, 24*(2)207–217. Retrieved from http://www.cell.com/cell-chemical-biology/fulltext/S2451-9456%2816%2930478-0

142Majority of Indian doctors are vitamin D deficient: Dr. Sanjay Kalra.
(2016, July 1). *The Health Site,* Retrieved from http://www.thehealthsite.com/news/majority-of-indian-doctors-are-vitamin-d-deficient-dr-sanjay-kalra-ag0616/

143Khayyat, Y., & Suzan, A. (2015). Vitamin D Deficiency in Patients
with Irritable Bowel Syndrome: Does it Exist? *Oman Med Journal, 30*(2), 115–118. Retrieved from https://www.ncbi.nlm.nih.gov/pmc/articles/PMC4412886/

144Wilson, J. & Christensen, J. (2014, February 27). Nutrition labels getting a makeover. *CNN.com.* Retrieved from http://www.cnn.com/2014/02/27/health/nutrition-labels-changes/index.html

145Tachimoto, H., Mezawa, H., Segawa, T., Akiyama, N., Ida, H., & Urashima, M. (2016). Improved control of childhood asthma with low-dose, short-term vitamin D supplementation: a randomized, double-blind, placebo-controlled trial. *Allergy, 71*(7), 1001–1009. Retrieved from https://www.ncbi.nlm.nih.gov/pubmed/26841365

146Ghai, B., Bansal, D., Kanukula, R., Gudala, K., Sachdeva, N., Dhatt, S. S., & Kumar, V. (2017). Vitamin D supplementation in patients with chronic low back pain: An open label, single arm clinical trial. *Pain Physician, 20*(1), E99-E105. Retrieved from https://www.ncbi.nlm.nih.gov/pubmed/28072801

147Bozkurt, N. C., Cakal, E., Sahin, M., Ozkaya, E. C., Firat. H., & Delibasi, T. (2012).The relation of serum 25-hydroxyvitamin-D levels with severity of obstructive sleep apnea and glucose metabolism abnormalities. *Endocrine, 41*(3), 518–525. Retrieved from https://www.ncbi.nlm.nih.gov/pubmed/22246808

148Mokry, L. E., Ross, S., Morris, J. A., Manousaki, D., Forgetta, V., & Richards, J. B. (2016). Genetically decreased vitamin D and risk of Alzheimer disease. *Neurology, 87*(24), 2567–2574. Retrieved from https://www.ncbi.nlm.nih.gov/pmc/articles/PMC5207000/

149Cannell, J. (2013, December 10). Why does the Vitamin D Council recommend 5,000 IU/day? *Vitamin D Council.* Retrieved from https://www.vitamindcouncil.org/why-does-the-vitamin-d-council-recommend-5000-iuday/

150Tovey, A. (2017, May 22). How much vitamin D is needed to achieve optimal levels? *Vitamin D Council.* Retrieved from https://www.vitamindcouncil.org/how-much-vitamin-d-is-needed-to-achieve-optimal-levels/

151Heaney, R. P., Armas, L. A. G., & French, C. (2013). All-source basal vitamin D inputs are greater than previously thought and cutaneous inputs are smaller. *The Journal of Nutrition, 143*(5), 571—575. Retrieved from http://jn.nutrition.org/content/143/5/571.long

152I tested my vitamin D level. What do my results mean? (n.d.). *Vitamin D Council.* Retrieved from https://www.vitamindcouncil.org/i-tested-my-vitamin-d-level-what-do-my-results-mean/

153Serrano, M. A., Cañada, J., Moreno, J. C., & Gurrea, G. (2017). Solar ultraviolet doses and vitamin D in a northern mid-latitude. *Science of the Total Environment, 574,* 744–750. Retrieved from https://www.ncbi.nlm.nih.gov/pubmed/27664761

154Fuentes, V. (2017, March 7). How much sun is good for our health? *SINC: Biomedicine And Health: Public Health.* Retrieved from http://www.agenciasinc.es/en/News/How-much-sun-is-good-for-our-health

155How do I get the vitamin D my body needs? (n.d.). *Vitamin D Council.* Retrieved from https://www.vitamindcouncil.org/about-vitamin-d/how-do-i-get-the-vitamin-d-my-body-needs/

156Patwardhan, V. G., Mughal, Z. M., Padidela, R., Chiplonkar, S. A., Khadilkar, V. V., & Khadilkar, A.V. (2017). Randomized Control Trial assessing impact of increased sunlight exposure versus vitamin D supplementation on lipid profile in Indian vitamin D deficient men. *Indian Journal of Endocrinology and Metabolism, 21*(3), 393–398. Reteieved from https://www.ncbi.nlm.nih.gov/pmc/articles/PMC5434721/

157Tovey, A. (2016, October 21). Are oral vitamin D3 sprays as effective as capsules? *Vitamin D Council.* Retrieved from https://www.vitamindcouncil.org/are-oral-vitamin-d3-sprays-as-effective-as-capsules/

158Owens, D. J., Tang, J. C., Bradley, W. J., Sparks, A. S., Fraser, W. D., Morton, J. P., & Close, G. L. (2017). Efficacy of high-dose vitamin D supplements for elite athletes. *Medicine and Science in Sports and Exercise, 49*(2), 349-356. Retrieved from https://www.ncbi.nlm.nih.gov/pubmed/27741217

159Todd, J. J., McSorley, E. M., Pourshahidi, L. K., Madigan, S. M., Laird, E., Healy, M., & Magee, P. J. (2016). Vitamin D3 supplementation in healthy adults: a comparison between capsule and oral spray solution as a method of delivery in a wintertime, randomised, open-label, cross-over study. *British Journal of Nutrition, 116*(8), 1402–1408. Retrieved from https://www.ncbi.nlm.nih.gov/pubmed/?term=Vitamin+D3+supplementation+in+healthy+adults%3A+a+comparison+between+capsule+and+oral+spray+solution+as+a+method+of+delivery+in+a+wintertime%2C+randomised%2C+open-label%2C+cross-over+study.

160Sadat-Ali, M., Bubshait, D. A., Al-Turki, H. A., Al-Dakheel, D. A. & Al-Olayani, W. S. (2014). Topical delivery of vitamin D3: A randomized controlled pilot study. *International Journal of Biomedical Sciience, 10*(1), 21–24. Retrieved from https://www.ncbi.nlm.nih.gov/pmc/articles/PMC3976443/

161Am I getting too much vitamin D? (n.d.) *Vitamin D Council.* Retrieved from https://www.vitamindcouncil.org/about-vitamin-d/am-i-getting-too-much-vitamin-d/

162Vitamin D. (2013, November 01). Retrieved from http://www.may-oclinic.org/drugs-supplements/vitamin-d/safety/hrb-20060400

163Abbasnezhad, A., Amani, R., Hajiani, E., Alavinejad, P., Cheraghian, B., & Ghadiri, A. (2016). Effect of vitamin D on gastrointestinal symptoms and health-related quality of life in irritable bowel syndrome patients: a randomized double-blind clinical trial. *Neurogastroenterology & Motility, 28*(10), 1533–1544. Retrieved from https://www.ncbi.nlm.nih.gov/pubmed/27154424

164Shomon, M (2017, July 31). The TSH reference range: A guide for thyroid patients. Retrieved from https://www.verywell.com/tsh-thyroid-stimulating-hormone-reference-range-wars-3232912

165Persky, W. (2008, June 4). Poll About Thyroid Issues. Retrieved from http://www.perskyfarms.com/phpBB2/viewtopic.php?t=7783

166Farhangi, M. A., Keshavarz, S. A., Eshraghian, M., Ostadrahimi, A., & Saboor-Yaraghi, A. A. (2012). The effect of vitamin A supplementation on thyroid function in premenopausal women. *The Journal of the American College of Nutrition, 31*(4), 268–274. Retrieved from https://www.ncbi.nlm.nih.gov/pubmed/23378454

167. DePaolo, R. W., Abadie, V., Tang, F., Fehlner-Peach, H., Hall J. A., Wang, W., . . . Jabri, B. (2011). Co-adjuvant effects of retinoic acid and IL-15 induce inflammatory immunity to dietary antigens. *Nature, 471*(7337), 220–224. Retrieved from http://www.ncbi.nlm.nih.gov/pubmed/21307853

168Skrovanek, S., DiGuilio, K., Bailey, R., Huntington, W., Urbas, R., Mayilvaganan, B., . . . Mullin, J. M. (2014). Zinc and gastrointestinal disease. *World Journal of Gastrointestinal Pathophysiology, 5*(4),496–513.

Retrieved from https://www.ncbi.nlm.nih.gov/pmc/articles/PM-C4231515/

169Mercola, J. (2013, December 08). Magnesium—The Missing Link to Better Health. Retrieved from http://articles.mercola.com/sites/articles/archive/2013/12/08/magnesium-health-benefits.aspx

170Dai, Q., Shrubsole, M. J., Ness, R. M., Schlundt, D., Cai, Q., Smalley, W. E., . . .Zheng, W. (2007). The relation of magnesium and calcium intakes and a genetic polymorphism in the magnesium transporter to colorectal neoplasia risk. *The American Journal of Clinical Nutrition, 86*(3), 743–751. Retrieved from https://www.ncbi.nlm.nih.gov/pmc/articles/PMC2082111/

171firespringInt, (2013, November 15). Why is the wheat genome so complicated? Retrieved from http://coloradowheat.org/2013/11/why-is-the-wheat-genome-so-complicated/

172Ezkurdia, I., Juan, D., Rodriguez, J, M., Frankish, A., Diekhans, M., Harrow, J., . . . Tress, M. L. (2014). Multiple evidence strands suggest that there may be as few as 19 000 human protein-coding genes. *Human Molecular Genetics, 23*(22), 5866–5878. Retrieved from https://www.ncbi.nlm.nih.gov/pmc/articles/PMC4204768/

173What are single nucleotide polymorphisms (SNPs)? (2017, June 27). Retrieved from https://ghr.nlm.nih.gov/primer/genomicresearch/snp

174MTHFR genetic mutation – what it is and how it can affect you. (n.d.). Retrieved from https://stopthethyroidmadness.com/mthfr/

17523andMe. (n.d.). Retreived from https://www.23andme.com/

176Methylation and detox analysis from 23andMe results. (n.d.). Retreived from http://geneticgenie.org/

177Promethease. (n.d.). Retreived from https://promethease.com/

178Genetic reports for single nucleotide polymorphisms. (n.d.). Retrieved from https://livewello.com

179Welcome to codegen.eu. (n.d.). Retrieved from https://codegen.eu

180NutraHacker. (n.d.). Retrieved from https://www.nutrahacker.com

181Unlimit Your Life. (n.d.). Retrieved from https://www.infino.me

182Import your genomic data and receive a free genome report. (n.d.). Retrieved from https://www.enlis.com/import

183Connect your DNA and Stay healthy. (n.d.). Retrieved from https://geneknot.com

184Kressor, C. (2012, March 9). The little known (but crucial) difference between folate and folic acid. Retrieved from https://chriskresser.-com/folate-vs-folic-acid/

185The chemical secrets of the Mediterranean diet: High levels of magnesium help to reduce risk of strokes, diabetes and heart disease. (Updated 2016, December 8). Retrieved from http://www.dailymail.-co.uk/health/article-4011708/The-chemical-secrets-Mediterranean-diet-High-levels-magnesium-help-reduce-risk-strokes-diabetes-heart-disease.html

186Mazur, A., Maier, J. A., Rock, E., Gueux, E., Nowacki, W., & Rayssiguier, Y. (2007). Magnesium and the inflammatory response: potential physiopathological implications. *Archives of Biochemistry and Biophysics, 458*(1), 48–56. Retrieved from https://www.ncbi.nlm.nih.gov/pubmed/16712775

187Håkanson, R., & Sundler, F. (1991). Histamine-producing cells in the stomach and their role in the regulation of acid secretion. Scandinavian Journal of Gastroenterology. Supplement, 180, 88–94. Retrieved from https://www.ncbi.nlm.nih.gov/pubmed/2042038

188Nishio, A., Ishiguro, S., & Miyao, N. (1987). Specific change of histamine metabolism in acute magnesium-deficient young rats. *Drug Nutrient Interactions, 5*(2), 89-96. Retrieved from https://www.ncbi.nlm.nih.gov/pubmed/3111814

189Watanabe, T., Kitamura, Y., Maeyama, K., Got, S., Yamatodani, A. & Wada, H. (1981). Absence of increase of histidine decarboxylase activity in mast cell-deficient W/W mouse embryos before parturition. Procedings of the National Academy of Sciences 78(7), 4209-4212. Retrieved from http://www.google.com/url?sa=t&rct=j&q=&esrc=s&source=web&cd=4&cad=rja&uact=8&ved=0ahUKEwiDlu-0mYDVAhXLQCYKHc2cDFQQFgg6MAM&url=http%3A%2F%2Fwww.pnas.org%2Fcontent%2F78%2F7%2F4209.full.pdf&usg=AFQjCNE_EiV5S-Ry9f_NTNwW-pLDhWDHxnQ

190Forbes, E. E., Groschwitz, K., Abonia, J. P., Brandt, E. B., Cohen, E., Blanchard, C., . . .Hogan, S. P. (2008). IL-9– and mast cell–mediated intestinal permeability predisposes to oral antigen hypersensitivity. *The Journal of Experimental Medicine, 205*(4), 897. Retrieved from http://jem.rupress.org/content/205/4/897

191Mast cell disorders of the gastrointestinal tract. (n.d.). Retrieved from http://www.brighamandwomens.org/Departments_and_Services/me dicine/services/gastroenterology/gastroenterology-and-gi-surgery-advances/reducing-gastrointestinal-symptoms-using-mast-cell-disorder-identification-and-treatment.aspx

192Castells, M. (2016, April 27). Castells lab (Biographical Sketch). Retrieved from http://www.brighamandwomens.org/Research/depts/Medicine/Rheu matology/Labs/castells/default.aspx

193Scherber, R. M., & Borate, U. (2017, October 19). How we diagnose and treat systemic mastocytosis in adults. *British Journal of Haematolology, 180*(1), 11–23. Retrieved from http://onlinelibrary.wiley.com/doi/10.1111/bjh.14967/full

194Ung, K., Gillberg, R., Kilander, A., & Abrahamsson, H. (2000). Role of bile acids and bile acid binding agents in patients with collagenous colitis. *Gut, 46*(2), 170–175. Retrieved from https://www.ncbi.nlm.nih.gov/pmc/articles/PMC1727822/

195Fernandez-Bañares, F., Esteve, M., Salas, A., Forné, T. M., Espinos, J. C., Martín-Comin, J., & Viver, J. M. (2001). Bile acid malabsorption in microscopic colitis and in previously unexplained functional chronic diarrhea. *Digestive Diseases and Sciences, 46*(10), 2231–2238. Retrieved from https://www.ncbi.nlm.nih.gov/pubmed/11680602

196Rose, A. J., Berriel Díaz, M., Reimann, A., Klement, J., Walcher, T., Krones-Herzig, A., . . . Herzig, S. (2011). Molecular control of systemic bile acid homeostasis by the liver glucocorticoid receptor. *Cell Metabolism, 14*(1), 123–130. Retrieved from https://www.ncbi.nlm.nih.gov/pubmed/21723510

197Park, T., Cave, D., & Marshall, C. (2015). Microscopic colitis: A review of etiology, treatment and refractory disease. *World Journal of Gastroenterology, 21*(29), 8804–8810. Retrieved from https://www.ncbi.nlm.nih.gov/pmc/articles/PMC4528022/

198Lundåsen, T., Gälman, C., Angelin, B., & Rudling, M. (2006). Circulating intestinal fibroblast growth factor 19 has a pronounced diurnal variation and modulates hepatic bile acid synthesis in man. *Journal of Internal Medicine, 260*(6), 530–536. Retrieved from http://onlinelibrary.wiley.com/doi/10.1111/j.1365-2796.2006.01731.x/abstract;jsessionid=4E5ACF2849FA6ED6F13371A471CC820B.f03t01

199Nolan, J. D., Johnston, I. M., Pattni, S. S., Dew, T., Orchard, T. R., & Walters, J. R. (2015). Diarrhea in Crohn's disease: investigating the role of the ileal hormone fibroblast growth factor 19. *Journal of Crohns & Colitis, 9*(2), 125–131. Retrieved from https://www.ncbi.nlm.nih.gov/pubmed/25518063

200Walters, J. R. (2014). Bile acid diarrhoea and FGF19: new views on diagnosis, pathogenesis and therapy. *Nature Reviews for Gastroenterology and Hepatology, 11*(7), 426–534. Retrieved from https://www.ncbi.nlm.nih.gov/pubmed/24662279

201Walters, J. R. F., & Appleby, R. N. (2015). A variant of FGF19 for treatment of disorders of cholestasis and bile acid metabolism. *Annals of Translational Medicine, 3*(1), S7. Retrieved from https://www.ncbi.nlm.nih.gov/pmc/articles/PMC4437929/

202Dukowicz, A. C., Lacy, B. E., & Levine, G. M. (2007). Small intestinal bacterial overgrowth. *Gastroenterology & Hepatology, 3*(2), 112–122. Retrieved from https://www.ncbi.nlm.nih.gov/pmc/articles/PMC3099351/

203Siebecker, A. (n.d.). SIBO associated diseases. SIBO- Small Intestine Bacterial Overgrowth. Retrieved from http://www.siboinfo.com/associated-diseases.html

204Jarred Younger, J., Luke Parkitny, L., & McLain, D. (2014). The use of low-dose naltrexone (LDN) as a novel anti-inflammatory treatment for chronic pain. *Clinical Rheumatology, 33*(4), 451–459. Retrieved from https://www.ncbi.nlm.nih.gov/pmc/articles/PMC3962576/

205Reimer, C., Søndergaard, B., Hilsted, L., & Bytzer, P. (2009). Proton-pump inhibitor therapy induces acid-related symptoms in healthy volunteers after withdrawal of therapy. *Gastroenterology, 137*(1), 80-87. Retrieved from https://www.ncbi.nlm.nih.gov/pubmed/19362552

206 McColl, K. E. L., & Gillen, D. (2009). Evidence That Proton-Pump Inhibitor Therapy Induces the Symptoms it Is Used to Treat. *Gastroenterology, 137*(1), 20–22. Retrieved from http://www.gastrojournal.org/article/S0016-5085%2809%2900780-X/fulltext

207Sampathkumar, K., Ramalingam, R., Prabakar, A., & Abraham, A. (2013). Acute interstitial nephritis due to proton pump inhibitors. *Indian Journal of Nephrology23*(4), 304–307. Rerieved from https://www.ncbi.nlm.nih.gov/pmc/articles/PMC3741979/

208Fallahzadeh, M. K., Borhani Haghighi, A., & Namazi, M. R. (2010). Proton pump inhibitors: predisposers to Alzheimer disease? *Journal of Clinical Pharmacology and Theraputics, 35*(2), 125–126. Retrieved from https://www.ncbi.nlm.nih.gov/pubmed/20456731

209Haenisch, B., von Holt, K., Wiese, B., Prokein, J., Lange, C., Ernst, A., . . . Scherer, M. (2015). Risk of dementia in elderly patients with the use of proton pump inhibitors. *European Archhives of Psychiatry and Clinical Neuroscience. 265*(5), 419–428. Retrieved from https://www.ncbi.nlm.nih.gov/pubmed/25341874

210Cannell, J. (2011, September 07). Dear Dr Cannell: Vitamin D and acid reflux. Retrieved from https://www.vitamindcouncil.org/vitamin-d-and-acid-reflux-august-mailbag-pt-3/

211Rathod, J. (2017, September 18). Can the "sunshine vitamin" help cure GERD? Retrieved from https://www.sepalika.com/gerd/vitamin-d-acid-reflux/

212Eades, M. (2005, November 25). Heartburn cured. Retrieved from https://proteinpower.com/drmike/2005/11/25/heartburn-cured/

213Kandil, T. S., Mousa, A. A., El-Gendy, A. A., & Abbas, A.M. (2010). The potential therapeutic effect of melatonin in gastro-esophageal reflux disease. *BMC Gastroenterology, 10*, 7. Retrieved from https://www.ncbi.nlm.nih.gov/pmc/articles/PMC2821302/

214Klupińska, G., Wiśniewska-Jarosińska, M., Harasiuk, A., Chojnacki, C., Stec-Michalska, K., Błasiak J., . . . Chojnacki, J. (2006). Nocturnal secretion of melatonin in patients with upper digestive tract disorders. Journal of *Physioliology & Pharmacology, 57*(5), 41–50. Retrieved from https://www.ncbi.nlm.nih.gov/pubmed/17218759

215How to Wean Off PPIs and Why. (n.d.). Retrieved from http://how-totreatheartburn.com/how-to-wean-off-ppis-and-why/

216Editorial staff. (2016, October 9). Why do placebos work? Retrieved from http://www.cbsnews.com/news/why-do-placebos-work/

217Rankin, L. (2011, December 27). Can Positive Thinking Help You Heal? Retrieved from https://www.psychologytoday.com/blog/owning-pink/201112/can-positive-thinking-help-you-heal

218Peters, S. L., Biesiekierski, J. R., Yelland, G. W., Muir, J. G., & Gibson, P. R. (2014). Randomised clinical trial: gluten may cause depression in subjects with non-coeliac gluten sensitivity - an exploratory clinical study. *Alimentary Pharmacology and Therapeutrics, 39*(10), 1104–1112. Retrieved from http://onlinelibrary.wiley.com/doi/10.1111/apt.12730/full

219Carta, M. G., Hardoy, M. C., Boi, M. F., Mariotti, S., Carpiniello, B., & Usai, P. (2002). Association between panic disorder, major depressive disorder and celiac disease: a possible role of thyroid autoimmunity. *Journal of Psychosomatic Research53*(3), 789–793. Retrieved from https://www.ncbi.nlm.nih.gov/pubmed/12217453

220Kurina, L., Goldacre, M., Yeates, D., &Gill, L. (2001). Depression and anxiety in people with inflammatory bowel disease. *Journal of Epidemiology & Community Health, 55*(10), 716–720. Retrieved from https://www.ncbi.nlm.nih.gov/pmc/articles/PMC1731788/

221Smith, R. S. (1997). How your immune system causes depression: Immunological Evidence Supporting The Immune-Cytokine Model of Depression. Retrieved from http://www.cytokines-and-depression.com/chapter7.html

222Kresser, C. (2014, August 19). Is Depression a Disease—or a Symptom of Inflammation? Retrieved from https://chriskresser.com/is-depression-a-disease-or-a-symptom-of-inflammation/

223Berk, M., Williams, L. J., Jacka, F. N., O'Neil, A., Pasco, J. A., Steven Moylan, S., . . . Maes, M. (2013). So depression is an inflammatory disease, but where does the inflammation come from? *BMC Medicine 201311*(200). Retrieved from http://bmcmedicine.biomedcentral.com/articles/10.1186/1741-7015-11-200

224Kirsch, I. (2014). Antidepressants and the Placebo Effect. *Zeitschrift Fur Psychologie, 222*(3), 128–134. Retrieved from https://www.ncbi.nlm.nih.gov/pmc/articles/PMC4172306/

225Begley, S. (2010, January 28). Why Antidepressants Are No Better Than Placebos. Retrieved from http://www.newsweek.com/why-an-tidepressants-are-no-better-placebos-71111

226Inflammation: The real cause of all disease and how to reduce and prevent it. (n.d.) Retrieved from https://bodyecology.com/articles/in-flammation_cause_of_disease_how_to_prevent.php

227Powell, N. D., Sloan, E. K., Bailey, M.T., Arevalo, J. M. G., Miller, G. E., Chen, E., . . . Cole, S. W. (2013). Social stress up-regulates inflam-matory gene expression in the leukocyte transcriptome via β-adren-ergic induction of myelopoiesis. *Proceedings of the National Academy of Sciences of the United States of Aamerica, 110*(41), 16574–16579. Re-trieved from http://www.pnas.org/content/110/41/16574.full

228Chronic stress changes immune cell genes, leading to inflammation: Study. (2013, November 11). Retrieved from http://www.huffington-post.com/2013/11/07/chronic-stress-health-inflammation-genes_n_4226420.html

229Stress causes whole body deterioration. (2008, January 9). Retrieved from http://www.news-medical.net/news/2008/01/09/34154.aspx

230National Academies of Sciences, Engineering, and Medicine; Health and Medicine Division; Food and Nutrition Board; Committee on Food Allergies: Global Burden, Causes, Treatment, Prevention, and Public Policy; Stallings, V. A., & Oria, M. P. (Eds). (2017). Finding a path to safety in food allergy: Assessment of the global burden, causes, prevention, management, and public policy. Washington, D.C.: The National Academies of Sciences, Engineering, & Medicine. Retrieved from https://www.nap.edu/catalog/23658/finding-a-path-to-safety-in-food-allergy-assessment-of

231Scott, F. I., Horton, D. B., Mamtani, R., Haynes, K., Goldberg, D.S., Lee, D. Y., & Lewis, J. D. (2016). Administration of antibiotics to children before age 2 years increases risk for childhood obesity. *Gastroenterology, 151*(1), 120–129. Retrieved from http://www.gastrojournal.org/article/S0016-5085%2816%2900352-8/abstract

232Tutuian, R. (2010). Adverse effects of drugs on the esophagus. *Best Practice & Research: Clinical Gastroenterology, 24*(2), 91–97. Retrieved from https://www.ncbi.nlm.nih.gov/pubmed/20227023

233Papapoulos, S. E. (2008). Bisphosphonates: how do they work? *Best Practice & Research: Clinical Endocrinolology & Metabolism, 22*(5), 831–847. Retrieved from https://www.ncbi.nlm.nih.gov/pubmed/19028359

234De Petris, G., Caldero, S. G., Chen, L., Xiao, S. Y., Dhungel, B. M., Spizcka, A. J., & Lam-Himlin, D. (2014). Histopathological changes in the gastrointestinal tract due to medications: an update for the surgical pathologist (part II of II). *International Journal of Surgical Pathology, 22*(3), 202–211. Retrieved from

https://www.ncbi.nlm.nih.gov/pubmed/24021900

235Parfitt, J. R., & Driman, D. K. (2007). Pathological effects of drugs on the gastrointestinal tract: a review. *Human Pathology, 38*(4), 527–536. Retrieved from https://www.ncbi.nlm.nih.gov/pubmed/17367604

236Wallace, J. L. (1997). Nonsteroidal anti-inflammatory drugs and gastroenteropathy: the second hundred years. *Gastroenterology, 112*(3), 1000–1016. Retrieved from https://www.ncbi.nlm.nih.gov/pubmed/9041264

237Nordqvist, C. (2011, August 24). Proton pump inhibitors should have black-box warnings, group tell FDA. Retrieved from https://www.medicalnewstoday.com/articles/233272.php

238FDA reminder to avoid concomitant use of Plavix (clopidogrel) and omeprazole – LECOM Education System. (2016, November 5). Retrieved from https://lecom.edu/fda-reminder-to-avoid-concomitant-use-of-plavix-clopidogrel-and-omeprazole/

239Lazarus, B., Chen, Y., & Wilson, F. P. (2016). Proton pump inhibitor use and the risk of chronic kidney disease. JAMA Internal Medicine, 176(2), 238–246. Retrieved from http://jamanetwork.com/journals/jamainternalmedicine/fullarticle/2481157

240Masclee, G. M., Coloma, P. M., Kuipers, E. J., & Sturkenboom, M. C. (2015). Increased risk of microscopic colitis with use of proton pump inhibitors and non-steroidal anti-inflammatory drugs. *American Journal of Gastroenterology, 110*(5), 749–759. Retrieved from https://www.ncbi.nlm.nih.gov/pubmed/25916221

aw, E. L., Badowski, M., Hung, Y.-T., Weems, K., Sanchez, A., & Lee, T. A. (2017). Association between proton pump inhibitors and microscopic colitis. *Annals of Pharmacotherapy, 51*(3), 253–63. Retrieved from http://journals.sagepub.com/doi/pdf/10.1177/1060028016673859

242Kendrick, M. (2016, September 21). What causes heart disease part XXI. Retrieved from https://drmalcolmkendrick.org/2016/09/21/what-causes-heart-disease-part-xxi/

243Shah, N. H., LePendu, P., Bauer-Mehren, A., Ghebremariam, Y. T., Iyer, S. V., Marcus, J., . . . Leeper, N. J. (2015). Proton pump inhibitor usage and the risk of myocardial infarction in the general population. *PLoS ONE, 10*(6): e0124653. Retrieved from http://journals.plos.org/plosone/article?id=10.1371/journal.pone.0124653

244Cooke, J. P., and Ghebremariam, Y. T. (2011). DDAH Says NO to ADMA. *Arteriosclerosis, thrombosis, and vascular biology, 31*, 1462-1464. Retrieved from http://atvb.ahajournals.org/content/31/7/1462.full

245Freeman, H. J. (2008). Proton pump inhibitors and an emerging epidemic of gastric fundic gland polyposis. *World Journal of Gastroenterology 14*(9), 1318–1320. Retrieved from https://www.ncbi.nlm.nih.gov/pmc/articles/PMC2693675/

246Hagiwara, T., Mukaisho, K., Nakayama, T., Hattori, T., & Sugihara, H. (2015). Proton pump inhibitors and helicobacter pylori-associated pathogenesis. *Asian Pacific Journal of Cancer Prevention, 16*(4), 1315–1319. Retrieved from https://www.ncbi.nlm.nih.gov/pubmed/25743791

247Rubio-Tapia, A., Herman, M. L., Ludvigsson, J. F., Kelly, D. G., Mangan, T.F., Wu, T-T., & Murray, J. A. (2012). Severe Spruelike Enteropathy Associated With Olmesartan. *Mayo Clinic Proceedings, 87*(8), 732–738. Retrieved from https://www.ncbi.nlm.nih.gov/pmc/articles/PMC3538487/

248Allison, M. C., Howatson, A. G., Torrance, C. J., Lee, F. D., & Russell, R. I. (1992). Gastrointestinal Damage Associated with the Use of Nonsteroidal Antiinflammatory Drugs. *The New England Journal of Medicine, 327*, 749–754. Retrieved from http://www.nejm.org/doi/full/10.1056/NEJM199209103271101#t=article

249Bonagura, G. A., Ribaldone, D. G., Fagoonee, S., Sapone, N., Caviglia, G. P., Saracco, G. M., . . . Pellicano, R. (2016). Microscopic colitis in patients with mild duodenal damage: A new clinical and pathological entity ("lymphocytic enterocolitis")? *World Journal of Gastrointestestianl Pathophysiology, 7*(4), 307–313. Retrieved from https://www.ncbi.nlm.nih.gov/pmc/articles/PMC5108976/

250Celiac Disease: Digestive and Liver Health: University of Michigan Medicine. Retrieved from http://www.uofmhealth.org/conditions-treatments/digestive-and-liver-health/celiac-disease

251Northwestern Medicine: Gastroenterology Behavioral Medicine Program. Retrieved from https://www.nm.org/conditions-and-care-areas/digestive-health/gastroenterology-behavioral-medicine-program

252Dolhun, R. (2014, December 08). Gut check on Parkinson's: New findings on bacteria levels. Retrieved from https://www.michaeljfox.org/foundation/news-detail.php?gut-check-on-parkinson-new-findings-on-bacteria-levels ınaisas, S., Maher, J., & Kanthasamy, A. (2016). Gut microbiome in health and disease: Linking the microbiome-gut-brain axis and environmental factors in the pathogenesis of systemic and neurodegenerative diseases. *Pharmacology & Therapeutics, 158*, 52–62. Retrieved from https://www.ncbi.nlm.nih.gov/pmc/articles/PMC4747781/

254Golts, N., Snyder, H., Frasier, M., Theisler, C., Choi, P., & Wolozin, B. (2002). Magnesium inhibits spontaneous and iron-induced aggregation of alpha-synuclein. *Journal of Biological Chemistry, 277*(18), 16116–16123. Retrieved from http://www.jbc.org/content/277/18/16116.long

255Butler, M. W., Burt, A., Edwards, T. L., Zuchner, S., Scott, W. K., Martin, E. R., . . . Wang, L. (2011). Vitamin D receptor gene as a candidate gene for Parkinson disease. *Annals of Human Genetics, 75*(2), 201–210. Retrieved from https://www.ncbi.nlm.nih.gov/pmc/articles/PM-C3077063/

256Zhao, Y., Sun, Y., Ji, H. F., & Shen, L. (2013). Vitamin D levels in Alzheimer's and Parkinson's diseases: a meta-analysis. *Nutrition, 29*(6), 828–832. Retrieved from https://www.ncbi.nlm.nih.gov/pubmed/23415143

257Barbaro, M. R., Cremon, C., Caio, G., De Giorgio, R., Volta, U., Stanghellini, V., & Barbara, G. (2015). 247 Zonulin serum levels are increased in non-celiac gluten sensitivity and irritable bowel syndrome with diarrhea. *Gastroenterology, 148*(4), Supplement 1, Page S-56. Retrieved from http://www.gastrojournal.org/article/S0016-5085%2815%2930192-X/abstract

258MacDonald, F. (2017, January 3). It's official: A brand-new human organ has been classified. Retrieved from https://www.sciencealert.-com/it-s-official-a-brand-new-human-organ-has-been-classified

259Sideri, A., Bakirtzi, K., Shih, D. Q., Koon, H. W., Fleshner, P. Arsenescu, R. . . . Pothoulakis, C. (2015). Substance P mediates proinflammatory cytokine release from mesenteric adipocytes in inflammatory bowel disease patients. *Cellular and Molecular Gastroenterology and Hepatology, 1*(4), 420–432. Retrieved from https://www.ncbi.nlm.nih.gov/pmc/articles/PMC4629258/

260Halfvarson, J., Brislawn, C. J., Lamendella, R., Vázquez-Baeza, Y., Walters, W. A., Bramer, L. M., . . . Jansson, J. K. (2017, Feruary 13). Dynamics of the human gut microbiome in inflammatory bowel disease. *Nature Microbiology, 7*(17004). Advance online publication. Retrieved from http://www.nature.com/articles/nmicrobiol20174#abstract

261Suskind, D. L., Cohen, S. A., Brittnacher, M. J., Wahbeh, G., Lee, D., Shaffer, M. L., . . . Miller, S. I. (2016). Clinical and fecal microbial changes with diet therapy in active inflammatory bowel disease. *Journal of Clinical Gastroenterology, 52*(2), 155–163. Retrieved from https://www.ncbi.nlm.nih.gov/pubmed/28030510

262Novel diet shows promise in treating children with Crohn's disease and ulcerative colitis. (2016, Dec 28). Retrieved from http://www.prnewswire.com/news-releases/novel-diet-shows-promise-in-treating-children-with-crohns-disease-and-ulcerative-colitis-300383912.html

263Wong, A. P., Clark, A. L., E.A., Acree, M., Cohen, S.A., Ferry, G. D., & Heyman, M. B. (2009). Use of complementary medicine in pediatric patients with inflammatory bowel disease: Results from a multicenter survey. *Journal of Pediatric Gastroenterology and Nutrition, 48*(1), 55–60. Retrieved from https://www.ncbi.nlm.nih.gov/pmc/articles/PMC3250599/

̵ünch, A., Bohr, J., Miehlke, S., Benoni, C., Olesen, M., Öst, Å., . . . Ström, M. (2016). Low-dose budesonide for maintenance of clinical remission in collagenous colitis: a randomised, placebo-controlled, 12-month trial *Gut, 65*, 47–56. Retrieved from http://gut.bmj.com/content/65/1/47

265Staff. (2015, May 27). Patients who receive steroids for IBD At heightened risk for diabetes. Gastroenterology & Endoscopy News. Retrieved from http://www.gastroendonews.com/In-the-News/Article/05-15/Patients-Who-Receive-Steroids-for-IBD-At-Heightened-Risk-for-Diabetes/32422/ses=ogst

266Phan, T. X., Jaruga, B., Pingle, S. C., Bandyopadhyay, B. C., & Ahern, G. P. (2016). Intrinsic Photosensitivity Enhances Motility of T Lymphocytes. *Scientific Reports, 6*, 39479. Retrieved from http://www.nature.com/articles/srep39479

267Nguyen, G. C., Smalley, W. E., Vege, S. S., Carrasco-Labra, A. & the Clinical Guidelines Committee. (2016, December 18). American Gastroenterological Association Institute guideline on the medical management of microscopic colitis. *Gastroenterology, 150*, 242–246. Retrieved from http://www.gastrojournal.org/article/S0016-5085(15)01625-X/pdf

268Wild, D. (2016, March 21). Probiotic Effective for IBS and Eradicates SIBO. Gastroenterology & Endoscopy News. Retrieved from http://www.gastroendonews.com/In-the-News/Article/03-16/Probiotic-Effective-for-IBS-and-Eradicates-SIBO/35500/ses=ogst

269Gray, S. L., Anderson, M. L., Dublin, S., Hanlon, J. T., Hubbard, R., Walker, R., Yu O., . . . Larson, E. B. (2015). Cumulative use of strong anticholinergics and incident dementia: a prospective cohort study.

JAMA Internal Medicine, 175(3), 401–407. Retrieved from https://ja-manetwork.com/journals/jamainternalmedicine/fullarticle/2091745

270(2016, January 11). Targeted Immuno Therapies AB and Ferring Pharmaceuticals sign a strategic collaboration agreement for the treatment of IBD. Retrieved from https://www.ferring.com/en/media/press-releases/tla-and-fer-ring-sign-strategic-collaboration-for-the-treatment-of-ibd-11-jan-2016/

271(n.d.). Tailored Leukapheresis Treatment. Immune Therapy Hold-ings. Retrieved from http://ithgroup.eu/tailored-leukapheresis

272Hawkey, C. J., Snowden, J. A., Lobo, A., Belinger, C., & Tyndall, (2000). A. Stem cell transplantation for inflammatory bowel disease: practical and ethical issues, *Gut (2000)*46, 869–872. Retrieved from http://gut.bmj.com/content/46/6/869

273Flores, A. I., Gómez-Gómez, G. J., Masedo-González, Á. & Martínez-Montiel, M. P. (2015).Stem cell therapy in inflammatory bowel dis-ease: A promising therapeutic strategy? *World Journal of Stem Cells,7*(2), 343–351. Retrieved from https://www.ncbi.nlm.nih.gov/pmc/articles/PMC4369491/

274Dhayakaran, R., Neethirajan, S., & Weng, X. (2016). Investigation of the antimicrobial activity of soy peptides by developing a high throughput drug screening assay. *Biochemistry and Biophysics Reports, 2016*(6), 149–157. Retrieved from https://www.ncbi.nlm.nih.gov/pmc/articles/PMC5600318/

275Bueckert, K. (2016, April 26).Soy can be used as an antibacterial agent to fight food-borne illnesses, University of Guelph study finds

log message]. CBCNews. Retrieved from
.tp://www.cbc.ca/news/canada/kitchener-waterloo/universi-
ty-guelph-soybeans-inhibit-microbial-pathogens-1.3552120

276Meng, Q., Ying, Z., Noble, E., Zhao, Y., Agrawal, R., Mikhail, A., . . .
Yang, X. (2016). Systems nutrigenomics reveals brain gene networks
linking metabolic and brain disorders. *EBioMedicine, 2016*(7), 157–166.
Retrieved from http://www.ebiomedicine.com/article/S2352-
3964%2816%2930143-8/fulltext?cc=y=

277Wolpert, S. (2016, April 21). Fructose alters hundreds of brain genes,
which can lead to a wide range of diseases. Retrieved from
http://newsroom.ucla.edu/releases/fructose-alters-hundreds-of-brain-
genes-which-can-lead-to-a-wide-range-of-diseases

278Tabbaa, M., Golubic, M., Roizen, M. F., & Bernstein, A. M. (2013). Docosahexaenoic acid, inflammation, and bacterial dysbiosis in relation
to periodontal disease, inflammatory bowel disease, and the metabolic syndrome. *Nutrients, 5*(8), 3299–3310. Retrieved from
https://www.ncbi.nlm.nih.gov/pmc/articles/PMC3775255/

279Liu, H., Huang, D., McArthur, D. L., Boros, L. G., Nissen, N., &
Heaney, A. P. (2010). Fructose induces transketolase flux to promote
pancreatic cancer growth. *Cancer Research, 79*(15), 6,368–6,376. Retrieved from
http://cancerres.aacrjournals.org/content/70/15/6368.long

280Elliott, S.S., Keim, N. L., Stern, J. S., Teff, K., & Havel, P. J. (2002).
Fructose, weight gain, and the insulin resistance syndrome. The
American Journal of Clinical Nutriton, 76(5), 911–922. Retrieved from
http://ajcn.nutrition.org/content/76/5/911.full

281Ma, J., Jacques, P. F., Meigs, J. B., Fox, C. S., Rogers, G. T., Smith, C. E., . . . McKeown, N. M. (2016). Sugar-sweetened beverage but not diet soda consumption is positively associated with progression of insulin resistance and prediabetes. *The Journal of Nutrition, 146*(12), 44–2550. Retrieved from https://www.ncbi.nlm.nih.gov/pubmed/27934644

282Thompson, D. (2016, November 10). Daily Can of Soda Boosts Odds for Prediabetes, Study Finds. Health Day News. Retrieved from https://consumer.healthday.com/diseases-and-conditions-informa-tion-37/prediabetes-995/daily-can-of-soda-boosts-odds-for-predia-betes-study-finds-716755.html

283Moreno, M. L., Cebolla, Á., Muñoz-Suano, A., Carrillo-Carrion, C., Comino, I., Pizarro, Á., . . . Sousa, C. (2017). Detection of gluten im-munogenic peptides in the urine of patients with coeliac disease re-veals transgressions in the gluten-free diet and incomplete mucosal healing. *Gut, 66*(2), 250–257. Retrieved from https://www.ncbi.nlm.ni-h.gov/pmc/articles/PMC5284479/

284Karatzas, P. S., Gazouli, M., Safioleas, M., & Mantzarisa, G. J. (2014). DNA methylation changes in inflammatory bowel disease. *Annals of Gastroenterology, 27*(2), 125–132. Retrieved from https://www.ncbi.nlm.nih.gov/pmc/articles/PMC3982627/

285Cheung, K. S., Chan, E. W., Wong, A. Y. S., Lijia Chen, L., Wong, I. C. K., & Leung, W. K. (2017). Long-term proton pump inhibitors and risk of gastric cancer development after treatment for Helicobacter pylori: A population-based study. *Gut.* Advance online publication. Retrieved from http://gut.bmj.com/content/early/2017/09/18/gutjnl-2017-314605

za, R. F., Huo, X., Mittal, V., Schuler, C. M., Carmack, S. W., nang, H. Y., & Spechler, S. J. (2009). Gastroesophageal reflux might cause esophagitis through a cytokine-mediated mechanism rather than caustic acid injury. Gastroenterology, 137(5), 1776–1784. Retrieved from http://www.gastrojournal.org/article/S0016-5085%2809%2901378-X/abstract

287Dunbar, K. B., Agoston, A. T., & Odze, R.D. (2016). Association of acute gastroesophageal reflux disease with esophageal histologic changes. JAMA, 315(19), 2104-2112. Retrieved from https://jamanetwork.com/journals/jama/fullarticle/2521970

288Chu, H., Khosravi, A., Kusumawardhani, I. P., Kwon, A. H. K., Vasconcelos, A. C., Cunha, L. D., . . . Mazmanian, S. K. (2016). Gene-microbiota interactions contribute to the pathogenesis of inflammatory bowel disease. Science, 352(6289), 1116–1120. Retrieved from http://science.sciencemag.org/content/352/6289/1116

289Manios, Y., Moschonis, G., Lambrinou, C. P., Tsoutsoulopoulou, K., Binou, P., Karachaliou, A., . . . Cashman, K. D. (in press). A systematic review of vitamin D status in southern European countries. European Journal of Nutrition, [Epublication ahead of print]. 2017, Cctober 31. Retrieved from https://www.ncbi.nlm.nih.gov/pubmed/29090332

290Vukman, K. V., Lalor, R., Aldridge, A., & O'Neill, S. M. (2016). Mast cells: New therapeutic target in helminth immune modulation. Parasite Immunology, 38(1). 45–52. Retrieved from https://www.ncbi.nlm.nih.gov/pubmed/26577605

291Rajamani, U., Gross, A. R., Ocampo, C., Andres, A. M., Gottlieb, R. A., & Sareen, D. (2017). Endocrine disruptors induce perturbations in endoplasmic reticulum and mitochondria of human pluripotent stem cell derivatives. *Nature Communications, 8*(Article number: 219). Retrieved from http://www.nature.com/articles/s41467-017-00254-8

292Ruiz, P. A., Morón, B., Becker, H. M., Lang, S., Atrott, K., Spalinger, M. R., . . . Rogler, G. (2017). Titanium dioxide nanoparticles exacerbate DSS-induced colitis: Role of the NLRP3 inflammasome. *Gut, 66*(7), 1216–1224. Retrieved from http://gut.bmj.com/content/66/7/1216

293Tan, J., McKenzie, C., Vuillermin, P. J., Goverse, G., Vinuesa, C. G., Mebius, R. E., . . . Mackay, C. R. (2016). Dietary fiber and bacterial SCFA enhance oral tolerance and protect against food allergy through diverse cellular pathways. *Cell Reports, 15*(12), 2809–2824. Retrieved from http://www.cell.com/cell-reports/fulltext/S2211-1247(16)30630-1?_returnURL=http%3A%2F%2Flinkinghub.elsevier.-com%2Fretrieve%2Fpii%2FS2211124716306301%3Fshowall%3Dtrue

294Oittinen, M., Popp. A., Kurppa, K., Lindfors, K., Mäki, M., Kaikkonen, M., & Viiri, K. (2017).Polycomb Repressive Complex 2 Enacts Wnt Signaling in Intestinal Homeostasis and Contributes to the Instigation of Stemness in Diseases Entailing Epithelial Hyperplasia or Neoplasia. *Stem Cells, 35*(2), 445–457. Retrieved from https://www.ncbi.nlm.nih.gov/pubmed/27570105

295Kandil, T. S., Mousa, A. A., El-Gendy, A. A., & Abbas, A. M. (2010). The potential therapeutic effect of melatonin in gastro-esophageal reflux disease. *BMC Gastroenterology, 10,* 7 Retrieved from https://www.ncbi.nlm.nih.gov/pmc/articles/PMC2821302/

296de Oliveira Torres, J. D. F., & de Souza Pereira, R. (2010). Which is the best choice for gastroesophageal disorders: Melatonin or proton pump inhibitors? *World Journal of Gastrointestinal Pharmacology and rapeutics, 1*(5), 102–106. Retrieved from https://www.ncbi.nlm.nih.gov/pmc/articles/PMC3091156/

297Esteve, M., Mahadevan, U., Sainz, E., Rodriguez, E., Salas, A., & Fernández-Bañares, F. (2011). Efficacy of anti-TNF therapies in refractory severe microscopic colitis. *Journal of Crohn's and Colitis, 5*(6), 612–618. Retrieved from https://www.ncbi.nlm.nih.gov/pubmed/22115383

298Park, T., Cave, D., & Marshall, C. (2015). Microscopic colitis: A review of etiology, treatment and refractory disease. *World Journal of Gastroenterology, 21*(29), 8804–8810. Retrieved from https://www.ncbi.nlm.nih.gov/pmc/articles/PMC4528022/

299Belyaev, I., Dean, A., Eger, H., Hubmann, G., Jandrisovits, R., Kern, M., . . . Thill, R. (2016). EUROPAEM EMF Guideline 2016 for the prevention, diagnosis and treatment of EMF-related health problems and illnesses. *Reviews on Environmental Health, 31*(3), 363–397. Retrieved from https://www.ncbi.nlm.nih.gov/pubmed/27454111

300Kabbani, T. A., Koutroubakis, E., Schoen, R. E., Ramos-Rivers, C., Shah, N., Swoger, J., . . . Binion, D. G. (2016). Association of vitamin D level with clinical status in inflammatory bowel disease: A 5-year longitudinal study. *The American Journal of Gastroenterology, 111*(5), 712–719. Retrieved from https://www.ncbi.nlm.nih.gov/pubmed/26952579

301Meier, H. C., Sandler, D. P., Simonsick, E. M., & Parks, C. G. (2016). Association between vitamin D deficiency and antinuclear antibodies in middle-aged and older U.S. adults. *Cancer Epidemiology, Biomarkers & Prevention, 25*(12), 1559–1563. Retrieved from https://www.ncbi.nlm.nih.gov/pubmed/27543618

302Meeker, S., Seamons, A., Maggio-Price, L., & Paik, J. (2016). Protective links between vitamin D, inflammatory bowel disease and colon cancer. *World Journal of Gastroenterology, 22*(3), 933–948. Retrieved from https://www.ncbi.nlm.nih.gov/pmc/articles/PMC4716046/

303Garland, C. F., & Gorham, E. D. (2017). Dose-response of serum 25-hydroxyvitamin D in association with risk of colorectal cancer: A meta-analysis. *Journal of Steroid Biochemistry and Molecular Biology, 168*(1),1-8. Retrieved from https://www.ncbi.nlm.nih.gov/pubmed/27993551?dopt=Abstract

304Schöttker, B., Haug, U., Schomburg, L., Köhrle, J., Perna, L., Müller, H., . . . Brenner, H. (2013). Strong associations of 25-hydroxyvitamin D concentrations with all-cause, cardiovascular, cancer, and respiratory disease mortality in a large cohort study. *American Journal of Clinical Nutrition 97*(4), 782–793. Retrieved from http://ajcn.nutrition.org/content/97/4/782.long

305Gubatan, J., Mitsuhashi, S., Zenlea, T., Rosenberg, L., Robson, S., & Moss, A. C. (2017). Low serum vitamin D during remission increases risk of clinical relapse in patients with ulcerative colitis. *Clinical Gastroenterolory and Hepatology,15*(2), 240–246. Rerieved from https://www.ncbi.nlm.nih.gov/pubmed/27266980

306Panwar, A., Valupadas, C., Veeramalla, M., & Vishwas, H. N. (in press). Prevalence of vitamin D deficiency in chronic and subacute low back pain patients in India: a triple-arm controlled study. *Clinical Rheumatology*, Retrieved from https://www.ncbi.nlm.nih.gov/pubmed/28842760

307Hajjaj-Hassouni, N., Mawani, N., Allali, F., Rkain, H., Hassouni, K., Hmamouchi, I., & Dougados, M. (2017). Evaluation of vitamin D sta-

...n rheumatoid arthritis and its association with disease activity ...ross 15 countries: "The COMORA study". *International Journal of Rheumatology*, 5491676. Retrieved from https://www.ncbi.nlm.nih.gov/pmc/articles/PMC5471553/

308Miclea, A., Miclea, M., Pistor, M., Hoepner, A., Chan, A., & Hoepner, R. (2017). Vitamin D supplementation differentially affects seasonal multiple sclerosis disease activity. *Brain and Behavior, 7*(8), e00761. Retrieved from https://www.ncbi.nlm.nih.gov/pmc/articles/PMC5561321/

309Turer, E., McAlpine, W., Wang, K. W., Lu, T., Li, X., Tang M., . . . Beutler, B. (2017). Creatine maintains intestinal homeostasis and protects against colitis. *Proceedings of the National Academy of Sciences, 114*(7), E1273–E1281. Retrioved from https://www.ncbi.nlm.nih.gov/pmc/articles/PMC5321020/

310Lappe, J., Travers-Gustafson, D., Garland, C., Heaney, R., Recker R., & Watson, P. (2016, October 31). 3352: Vitamin D3 and calcium supplementation significantly decreases cancer risk in older women [Web log blog]. American Public Health Association, Retrieved from https://apha.confex.com/apha/144am/meetingapp.cgi/Paper/368368

311Lappe, J., Watson, P., Travers-Gustafson, D., Recker, R., Garland, C. Gorham E. . . . McDonnell, S. L. (2017). Effect of vitamin D and calcium supplementation on cancer incidence in older women: A randomized clinical trial. *JAMA, 317*(12), 1234–1243. Retrieved from https://www.ncbi.nlm.nih.gov/pubmed/28350929

312Moslehi, N., Vafa, M., Rahimi-Foroushani, A., & Golestan. B. (2012). Effects of oral magnesium supplementation on inflammatory markers in middle-aged overweight women. *Journal of Research in Medical*

Sciences, 17(7), 607–614. Retrieved from https://www.ncbi.nlm.nih.-gov/pmc/articles/PMC3685774/

313Satija, A., Bhupathiraju, S. N., Rimm, E. B., Spiegelman, D., Chiuve, S.E., Borgi, L., . . . Hu, F. G. (2016). Plant-based dietary patterns and incidence of type 2 diabetes in US men and women: Results from three prospective cohort studies. PLOS Medicine 13(6): e1002039. Retrieved from http://journals.plos.org/plosmedicine/article?id=10.1371/journal.pmed.1002039

314American Heart Association. (201 7, November 13). Plant based diet associated with less heart failure risk. Retrieved from https://news-room.heart.org/news/plant-based-diet-associated-with-less-heart-fail-ure-risk

315Lambert, J., &Vojdani, A. (2017). Correlation of tissue antibodies and food immune reactivity in randomly selected patient specimens. *Journal of Clinical & Cellular Immunology, 8*(5), 521. Retrieved from https://www.omicsonline.org/open-access/correlation-of-tissue-anti-bodies-and-food-immune-reactivity-in-randomly-selected-patien-t-specimens-2155-9899-1000521-94554.html

316Ramsden, C. E., Zamora, D., Majchrzak-Hong, S., Faurot, K. R., Broste, S. K., Frantz, R. P., . . . Hibbeln, J. R. (2016). Re-evaluation of the traditional diet-heart hypothesis: analysis of recovered data from Minnesota Coronary Experiment (1968-73). *BMJ 2016*(353), i1246. Retrieved from http://www.bmj.com/content/353/bmj.i1246

317Sacks, F. M., Lichtenstein, A. H., Wu, J. H. Y., Appel, L. J., Creager, M. A., Kris-Etherton, P. M., . . . Van Horn, L. V., On behalf of the American Heart Association. (2017, June 15). Dietary fats and cardiovascular disease: A presidential advisory from the American Heart Associ-

..ı. Retrieved from
.tp://circ.ahajournals.org/content/early/2017/06/15/CIR.00000000000
00510

318May, A. (2017, June 16). Coconut oil isn't healthy. It's never been healthy. Retrieved from https://www.usatoday.com/story/news/nation-now/2017/06/16/coconut-oil-isnt-healthy-its-never-been-healthy/402719001/

319Taubes, G. (2017, June 17). Vegetable oils, (Francis) Bacon, Bing Crosby, and The American Heart Association. Retrieved from http://gary-taubes.com/vegetable-oils-francis-bacon-bing-crosby-and-the-american-heart-association/

320Siri-Tarino, P. W., Sun, Q., Hu, F. B., & Krauss, R. M. (2010). Saturated fat, carbohydrate, and cardiovascular disease. The American Journal of Clinical Nutrition, 91(3), 502–509. Retrrieved from https://www.ncbi.nlm.nih.gov/pmc/articles/PMC2824150/

321Pimpin, L., Wu, J. H. Y., Haskelberg, H., Del Gobbo, L., & Mozaffarian, D. (2016). Is butter back? A systematic review and meta-analysis of butter consumption and risk of cardiovascular disease, diabetes, and total mortality. *PLoS One, 11*(6), e0158118. Retrieved from http://journals.plos.org/plosone/article?id=10.1371%2Fjournal.pone.0158118

322Dehghan, M., Mente, A., Zhang, X., Swaminathan, S., Wei Li, W., Mohan, V., . . . Yusuf, S., DPhil on behalf of the Prospective Urban Rural Epidemiology (PURE) study investigators. (2017. Associations of fats and carbohydrate intake with cardiovascular disease and mortality in 18 countries from five continents (PURE): a prospective cohort study. *The Lancet, 390*(10107), 2050–2062. Retrieved from www.thelancet.-

com/journals/lancet/article/PIIS0140-6736(17)32252-3/fulltext

323Sheldrick, G. (2017, January 24). HEALTH WARNING: Just ONE cheeseburger or pizza binge 'could alter your metabolism'. Express. Retrieved from http://www.express.co.uk/life-style/health/757750/Just-ONE-cheeseburger-or-pizza-binge-could-al-ter-your-metabolism

324Hernández, E. A., Kahl, S., Seelig, A., Begovatz, P., Irmler, M., Kupriyanova, Y., . . . Roden, M. (2017). Acute dietary fat intake initiates alterations in energy metabolism and insulin resistance. *The Journal of Clinical Investigation, 127*(2), 695–708. Retrieved from https://www.ncbi.nlm.nih.gov/pmc/articles/PMC5272194/

325Laugerette, F., Furet, J. P., Debard, C., Daira, P,, Loizon, E., Géloën, A., . . . Michalski, M. C. (2012). Oil composition of high-fat diet affects metabolic inflammation differently in connection with endotoxin receptors in mice. *American Journal of Physiology-Endocrinology and Metabolism, 302*(3), E374–386. Retrieved from https://www.ncbi.nlm.nih.-gov/pubmed/22094473

326Uhde, M., Ajamian,M., Caio, G., De Giorgio, R., Indart, A., Green, P. H., . . . Alaedini, A. (2016). Intestinal cell damage and systemic immune activation in individuals reporting sensitivity to wheat in the absence of coeliac disease. *Gut, 65*, 1930–1937. Retrieved from http://gut.bmj.com/content/65/12/1930

327Zong, G., Lebwohl, B., Hu, F., Sampson, L., Dougherty, L., Willett, W., . . . Sun, Q. (2017, March 09).Low gluten diets may be associated with higher risk of type 2 diabetes. American Heart Association Meeting Report Presentation 11. Retrieved from http://newsroom.-heart.org/news/low-gluten-diets-may-be-associated-with-higher-riskype-2-diabetes

8Choung, R. S., Unalp-Arida, A., Ruhl, C. E., Brantner, T. L., Everhart, J. E., & Murray, J. A. (2017). Less Hidden Celiac Disease But Increased Gluten Avoidance Without a Diagnosis in the United States. *Mayo Clinic Proceedings, 92*(1), 30–38. Retrieved from http://www.mayoclinicproceedings.org/article/S0025-6196%2816%2930634-6/fulltext

329Kieboom, B. C. T., Licher, S., Wolters, F. J., Ikram, M. K., Hoorn, E. J., Zietse R., . . . Ikram, M. A. (2017). Serum magnesium is associated with the risk of dementia. *Neurology, 89*(16), 16–722. Retrieved from https://www.ncbi.nlm.nih.gov/pubmed/28931641

330Colman, R. J., & Rubin, D. T. (2014). Fecal microbiota transplantation as therapy for inflammatory bowel disease: a systematic review and meta-analysis. *Journal of Crohn's and Colitis, 8*(12), 1569–1581. Retrieved from https://www.ncbi.nlm.nih.gov/pmc/articles/PMC4296742/

331Fasullo, M. J., Al-Azzawi, Y., & Abergel, J. (2017, July 19). Microscopic Colitis After Fecal Microbiota Transplant. *ACG Case Reports Journal, 4*, e87. Retrieved from https://www.ncbi.nlm.nih.gov/pmc/articles/PMC5519401/

332Tariq, R., Smyrk, T., Pardi, D. S., Tremaine, W. J., & Khanna, S. (2016). New-Onset Microscopic Colitis in an Ulcerative Colitis Patient After Fecal Microbiota Transplantation. *The American Journal of Gastroenterology, 111*(5), 751–752. Retrieved from https://mayoclinic.pure.elsevier.com/en/publications/new-onset-microscopic-colitis-in-an-ulcerative-colitis-patient-af

333Münch, A., Aust, D., Bohr, J., Bonderup, O., Fernández Bañarese, F., Hjortswang, H., . . . for the European Microscopic Colitis Group (EMCG). (2012). Microscopic colitis: Current status, present and future challenges: Statements of the European Microscopic Colitis Group. *Journal of Crohn's and Colitis, 6*(9), 932–945. Retrieved from https://www.sciencedirect.com/science/article/pii/S1873994612002565

334Yang, W. H., Heithoff, D. M., Aziz, P. V., Sperandio, M., Nizet, V., Mahan, M. J., & Marth, J. D. (2017). Recurrent infection progressively disables host protection against intestinal inflammation *Science, 358*(6370), eaao5610 Retrieved from http://science.sciencemag.org/content/358/6370/eaao5610

ces

Made in the USA
Las Vegas, NV
10 March 2024

87002865R00193